D0130520

A NEW YOU IN 21 DAYS

Jo Glanville-Blackburn

Quadrille

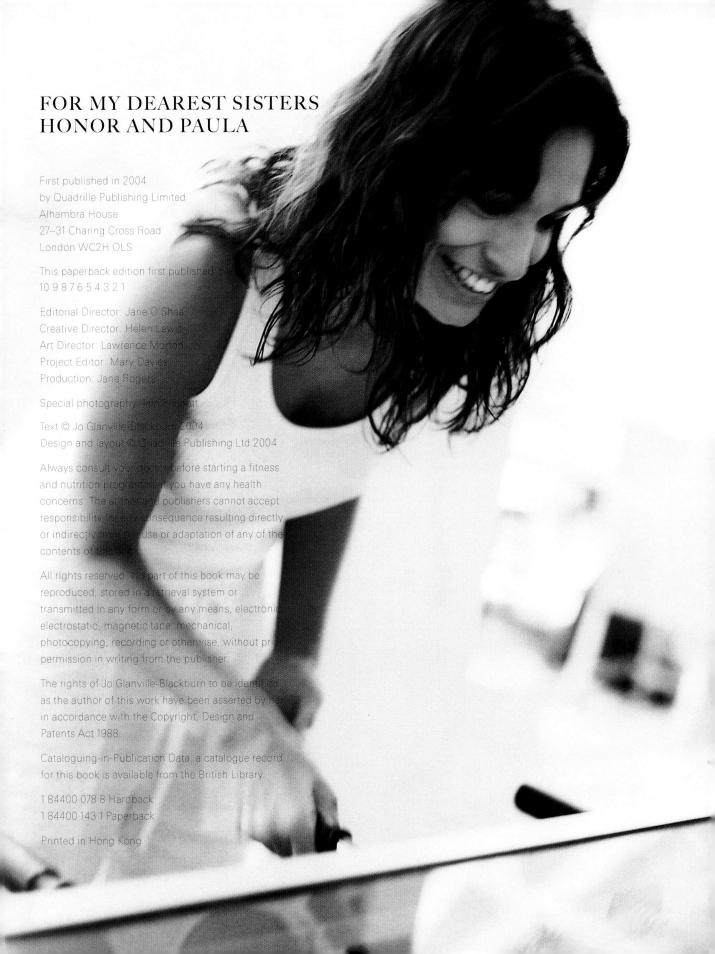

FOR MY DEAREST SISTERS HONOR AND PAULA

First published in 2004
by Quadrille Publishing Limited
Alhambra House
27–31 Charing Cross Road
London WC2H OLS

This paperback edition first published in
10 9 8 7 6 5 4 3 2 1

Editorial Director: Jane O'Shea
Creative Director: Helen Lewis
Art Director: Lawrence Morton
Project Editor: Mary Davies
Production: Jane Rogers

Special photography: Iain Hazlitt

Text © Jo Glanville-Blackburn 2004
Design and layout © Quadrille Publishing Ltd 2004

Always consult your doctor before starting a fitness
and nutrition programme if you have any health
concerns. The author and publishers cannot accept
responsibility for any consequence resulting directly
or indirectly from the use or adaptation of any of the
contents of this book.

All rights reserved. No part of this book may be
reproduced, stored in a retrieval system or
transmitted in any form or by any means, electronic,
electrostatic, magnetic tape, mechanical,
photocopying, recording or otherwise, without prior
permission in writing from the publisher.

The rights of Jo Glanville-Blackburn to be identified
as the author of this work have been asserted by her
in accordance with the Copyright, Design and
Patents Act 1988.

Cataloguing-in-Publication Data: a catalogue record
for this book is available from the British Library.

1 84400 078 8 Hardback
1 84400 143 1 Paperback

Printed in Hong Kong

Contents

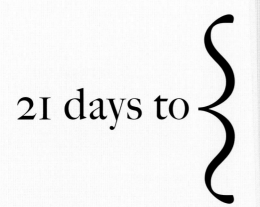

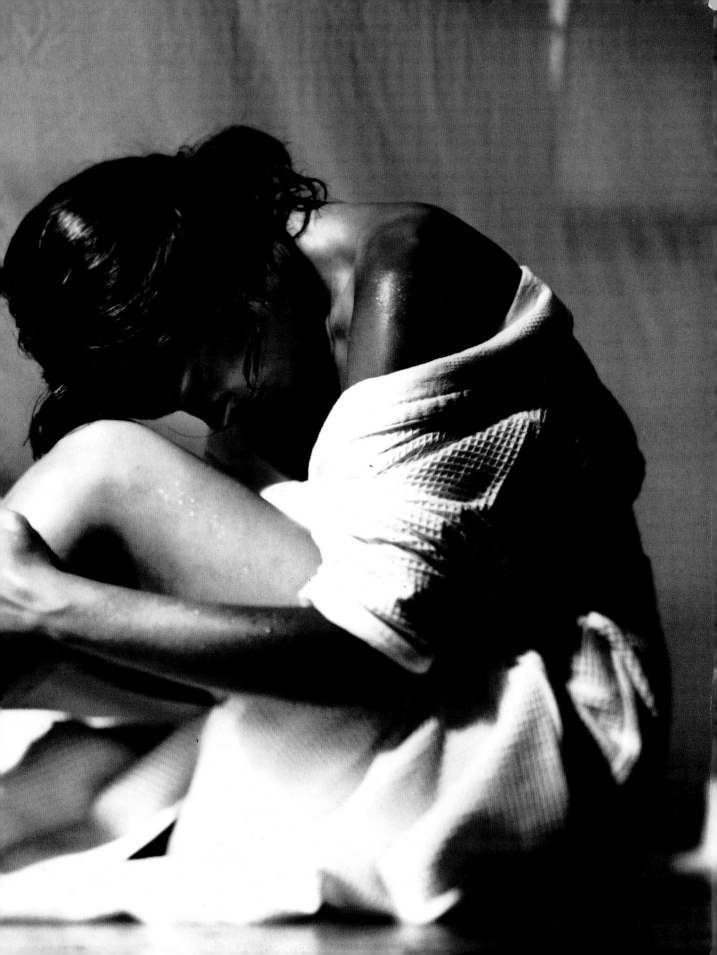

what is it about you?

So what would you like to improve? What are your goals? Glossier hair? A shapelier body? More energy? Better health? A calmer attitude? Well, you just have to focus on your strengths – and transform any weaknesses. Because there's no denying that you mirror the life that you lead. Your skin, hair and body reveal lifestyle pressures: stress, poor diet, insufficient sleep, lack of exercise and poor posture. And, ultimately, all lead to accelerated ageing and poor self-image.

How can anyone around us think the best of us if we don't do it for ourselves? Positive thinking is a therapy for every cell in your body. It's simply a way of directing your thoughts and feelings to find solutions to situations instead of allowing yourself to be held back by attitudes you established long ago.

It's time to become more aware of those self-limiting beliefs and the excuses you frequently make for yourself. How often do you just dismiss yourself as 'weak' or 'just not good enough'? Many self-belief issues run deep and can stem from your childhood, but they can and should be replaced by positive self-affirmations. I firmly believe that it is within our power to achieve the very best for ourselves. You can change anything if you want to.

Get yourself a notebook (you'll find that I recommend you keep one throughout the plan so you can monitor your progress) and begin with a list of all your strengths. Then make a list of your weaknesses, but set them down as positive goals – things you want to improve upon during this 21-day plan. Aim, in other words, for what you want to gain, not what you want to lose. Say, 'I want to become fit and healthy,' rather than, 'I want to lose weight.' Once you can hear and truly believe in the difference between those two statements, you will begin to see the difference...in you.

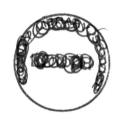

Accept yourself

Midlife crisis is an issue for many women today. Perhaps you gave up a career to have children and now, 15 years later, you find you've lost your sense of self and purpose in life. Perhaps you're going through a divorce and have lost all confidence to start over again, or maybe you've followed a lifelong career, chosen not to have a family, and suddenly find yourself made redundant.

Use this plan to change the way you think about yourself. You're sure to learn new tricks and techniques that make daily life more enjoyable. And you may even discover you relish some aspect – yoga,

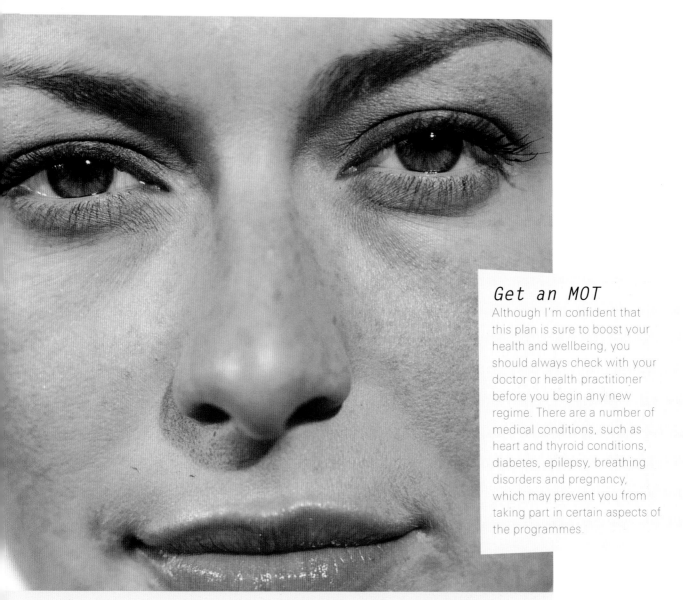

Get an MOT

Although I'm confident that this plan is sure to boost your health and wellbeing, you should always check with your doctor or health practitioner before you begin any new regime. There are a number of medical conditions, such as heart and thyroid conditions, diabetes, epilepsy, breathing disorders and pregnancy, which may prevent you from taking part in certain aspects of the programmes.

Care for yourself

aromatherapy, healthy eating, fitness – so much you take up a whole new interest that leads to a fresh career path. The only limitations are in you.

It's never too late, or too early, to start investing in yourself. Change your diet, bump up your fitness levels, take time out and indulge yourself. Looking good by looking after yourself isn't vanity – it's simply living the best you can for as long as you can. And, it's certain that, as you begin to feel better about yourself, you will demand less from yourself in negative ways, finding inner calm about who you are and what you want from your life.

Your body is forever sending out signals about your health and wellbeing. It's time to stop, look and listen. More than 80 per cent of visits to the doctor are stress related, from skin disorders, hair loss and high blood pressure to depression, heart disease and cancer, and that illustrates how so much of our health is in our own hands. Decide to neglect yourself no more. Monitor your body regularly so that if things do go out of sync you will be more aware of your normal reactions and better equipped to deal with change. This way you can help to keep your body looking and feeling its best for longer.

creating your own schedule

Over the next 21 days everything you do will make you look and feel like new. You'll learn how to take ten years off your skin, update your make-up, restyle your hair, reshape your body, eat for more energy and live a less stressful life. Some of the techniques you'll know already, but the real key to success is in making the programmes work for you and your lifestyle in the time that you have.

Understanding the plan

THIS 21-DAY PLAN IS DIVIDED INTO SEVEN PROGRAMMES (NUTRITION, FITNESS, SKINCARE, BODYCARE, MAKE-UP, HAIRCARE AND LOW STRESS) THAT WORK TOGETHER TO MAKE YOU LOOK AND FEEL LIKE NEW. THEY ARE BASED ON THREE ELEMENTS: DAILY, MUST-DO ROUTINES (TO FIT AROUND ANY WORK ROUTINE) THAT WILL <u>TRANSFORM</u> YOU, INSIDE AND OUT, AND EXTRAS TO FURTHER <u>BEAUTIFY</u> YOU AND <u>BOOST</u> YOUR MORALE AND ENERGY.

Turn the page and take a look at the sample planner for week one on pages 14–15. Everything not in script is a daily must – such as breakfast (don't skimp), exercise, and your skin and bodycare regimes. These are your

transformers

They are the daily essentials that will over these 21 days make a very real difference to the way you look and feel.

Next are the things that you can do whenever you have the time – once or in some instances more times a week (depending on your skin/hair type) – such as the blow-dry, facial mask, facial steam, scalp massage or body oil & salt scrub. These are the

beautifiers

They're not essential, but each one will help you look more groomed and gorgeous, and make you feel good about your body and much more in control of your life.

Finally there are the

boosters ☆

These are mind/body pick-me-ups – like the breathing ritual, life skills, manicure and pedicure, brow shaping and relaxing facial – to fit in as you feel you need them, significant rituals that will encourage you to devote extra time to yourself. All have a dramatic effect on your skin, hair, mind and body.

Making the plan work for you

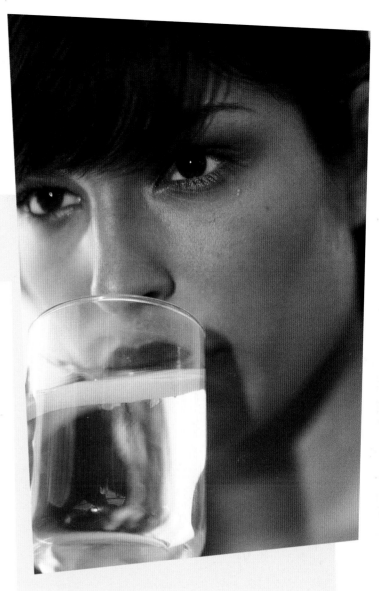

Focus on your needs You should fit the transformers in every day but which beautifiers and boosters you do is up to you. Read through the book, studying the age and lifestyle guides at the beginning of each programme, and noting down the beautifiers and boosters that most appeal to you and that best suit what you want to achieve. Then fill in your own weekly planner – there's a blank template printed on the inside back cover to photocopy. Finally, add any mind/body mini rituals to meet your own personal goals.

Make it your own The whole 21-day plan is designed to change the way you look and feel from top to toe, but you can tailor it to suit your special goals or the other demands on your time. If you're worried about your skin, then the Nutrition, Fitness, Skincare and Make-up chapters are for you. If you want to update your look, you need the Skincare, Make-up and Haircare chapters. If you want to downshift your stress levels, then concentrate on the Nutrition, Fitness and Low-Stress programmes.

Create your own timetable The times I have given on the sample planner on the next two pages, like the particular beautifiers and boosters I've chosen and highlighted, are only suggestions. I'm not about to tell you what time to get up or go to bed or how to organize your day. So choose time slots to suit your schedule. Just try to fit in as much as you can in the first week because you'll find yourself repeating many things in weeks two and three, and you'll get quicker as everything becomes more familiar.

Decide when to begin Start over a weekend, if you can, or when you have a couple of days free to really settle into the programme.

Plan ahead Buy the week's shopping – from fruit and vegetables to cotton wool, body scrub and aromatherapy oils – in advance. Make a checklist, using the essential kit at the start of each chapter and adding any special requirements for your personal choice of beautifiers and boosters.

Enjoy Take it gently, day by day, week by week, just immersing yourself in the sensation of truly looking after yourself. And give yourself little rewards at stages along the way: we all need encouragement!

your sample planner

THIS PLANNER SUGGESTS A POSSIBLE SCHEDULE FOR WEEK ONE OF THE 21-DAY PLAN FOR A WOMAN WORKING FULL TIME WHO HAS DECIDED TO FOLLOW ALL SEVEN PROGRAMMES. MUST-DO DAILY TRANSFORMER ROUTINES ARE SHOWN IN PRINT. THE OTHER ENTRIES (INDICATING TIMES, ♡BEAUTIFIERS AND ☆BOOSTERS) ARE HER CHOICE, AND THEY APPEAR IN SCRIPT SO THAT YOU CAN PICK THEM OUT QUICKLY.

Saturday		Sunday		Monday	
6.20am	Wake-up moments	7am	Wake-up moments	6.00am	Wake-up moments
6.30am	Early-morning stretch	7.10am	Early-morning stretch	6.20am	Early-morning stretch
6.50am	Body (am) regime	7.30am	*Mind power (visualization)* ☆	6.40am	*Feel-good stretch* ☆
7.00am	Skin (am) regime	7.50am	Body (am) regime	6.50am	Body (am) regime
	with facial steam ♡	8am	Skin (am) regime	7am	Skin (am) regime
7.15am	Hair regime		*with facial scrub* ♡	7.10am	Hair regime
7.25am	Breakfast	8.15am	Breakfast	7.20am	Breakfast
7.40am	*Scalp massage* ♡	8.45am	Hair regime	7.35am	Make-up *(am routine)*
7.50am	*Blow-dry* ♡				
	Energy treat		Energy treat		Energy treat
			Midday moments		*Time management* ☆
	Midday moments		Midday aerobics (walk)		Midday moments
	Lunch		Lunch		Lunch
	Mindpower (meditation) ☆		*Brow shaping* ☆		
	Pedicure ☆		*Snack*		*Snack*
	Snack		*Make-up update* ♡		
6.30pm	Evening tone-up			6.30pm	Evening tone-up
7pm	Supper	7pm	Supper	7pm	Supper
8.30pm	Body (pm) regime				
	with fake tan ☆	9pm	Body (pm) regime	9pm	Body (pm) regime
9pm	Skin (pm) regime	9.30pm	Skin (pm) regime	9.30pm	*Manicure* ☆
				10pm	Skin (pm) regime
10pm	Wind-down moments	10pm	Wind-down moments	10.20pm	Wind-down moments
	with breathing ritual ☆		*with breathing ritual* ☆		

Tuesday		Wednesday		Thursday		Friday	
6.00am	Wake-up moments	6am	Wake-up moments	6.00am	Wake-up moments	6am	Wake-up moments
6.20am	Early-morning stretch	6.20am	Early-morning stretch	6.20am	Early-morning stretch	6.20am	Early-morning stretch
6.40am	Body (am) regime	6.40am	Body (am) regime	6.40am	Body (am) regime	6.40am	Body (am) regime
6.50am	Skin (am) regime	6.50am	Skin (am) regime		*with oil & salt scrub* ♡	6.50am	Skin (am) regime
7am	Hair regime	7am	Hair regime	7am	Skin (am) regime		*with facial mask* ♡
				7.10am	Hair regime		
7.15am	Breakfast	7.15am	Breakfast	7.25am	Breakfast	7.15am	Breakfast
7.30am	*Blow-dry* ♡	7.30am	Make-up *(am routine)*	7.40am	Make-up *(fast track)*	7.30am	*Manicure* ☆
8am	Make-up *(am routine)*		*with lash curling* ☆				
	Energy treat		Energy treat		Energy treat		Energy treat
							Create order ☆
	Aromatherapy (energize) ☆		*Mind-power (games)* ☆		Midday moments		
	Midday aerobics (walk)		Midday moments		Midday aerobics (walk)		Midday aerobics (walk)
	Lunch		Lunch		Lunch		Lunch
	Midday moments		*Aromatherapy (calm)* ☆				Midday moments
	Snack		*Snack*		*Snack*		*Snack*
		6.30pm	Evening tone-up			6.30pm	Hair regime
7pm	Supper	7pm	Supper	7pm	Supper	7pm	Supper
				8.30pm	Body (pm) regime	7.30pm	Make-up (pm)
		9pm	*Mind power (meditation)* ☆	8.50pm	*Foot massage* ☆		
9.30pm	Body (pm) regime	9.30pm	Body (pm) regime	9.20pm	Skin (pm) regime	10.30pm	Body (pm) regime
9.50pm	Skin (pm) regime	9.50pm	Skin (pm) regime		*& anti-ageing massage* ☆	10.50pm	Skin (pm) regime
10pm	Wind-down moments	10pm	Wind-down moments	10pm	Wind-down moments	11pm	Wind-down moments
	with breathing ritual ☆				*with breathing ritual* ☆		*with breathing ritual* ☆

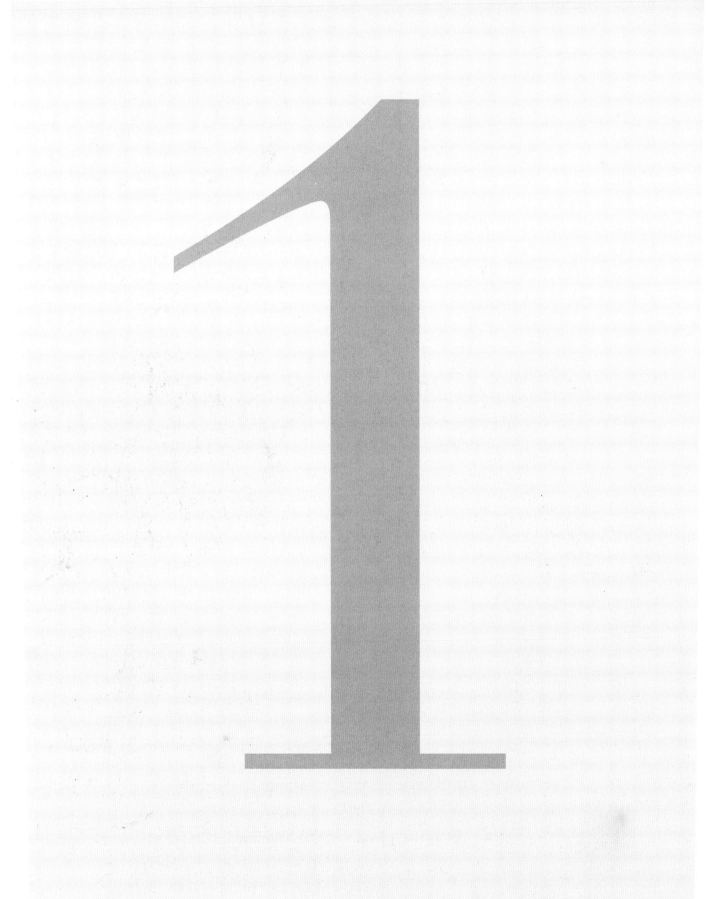

21 DAYS

TO

BETTER

EATING

Food is energy: pure energy for mind, body and soul. Fuel your body to a new level so you can live life to the full and achieve all you wish for in life.

Your nutrition programme

Follow this simple, tasty, healthy-eating plan based on food combining and energy-giving superfoods and you'll be amazed how much better nutrition reinforces almost every other aspect of your beauty and wellbeing. Did I say tasty? That's another perk in your new regime. If your diet has been heavily reliant on processed foods, prepare to witness the revival of your tastebuds.

THESE 21 DAYS ARE TURNAROUND TIME, SO JUST BE AWARE: EVERYTHING YOU PUT IN YOUR BODY SHOWS.

Why do we eat? Supplying your body with the nourishment it needs to support you – your body, your mind, your spirits – that's what food is about. Historically we come from a long line of meat eaters (I'm thinking cavemen here), but slowly we've evolved into a culture dependent largely on carbohydrates (the bulk of the highly tempting processed, pre-packed food we've invented for ourselves). And, as most nutrition experts would agree, our bodies can't cope. We simply haven't evolved in line with our diet.

What should we eat? A healthy, balanced diet makes sure you have enough energy and nutrients from every food group to thrive inside and out. We're talking superfoods (see page 35), raw or lightly cooked whole (that's unprocessed) foods, high in natural enzymes and phyto-chemicals, and wherever possible organic foods.

When you're tired or unhappy It's easy to get into the habit of using food as a stimulant to pick you up and keep you going. The way we live our lives now - too many processed foods and sugary snacks, endless cups of tea and coffee, frequent glasses of wine combined with high levels of stress (which makes us yearn for all of the above) – leads straight to toxic overload, and the result is that our bodies are as stressed as we are. And the classic signs of a body out of balance? They are tiredness, lethargy, spots, poor skin tone, poor digestion (constipation, diarrhoea and IBS), headaches, irritability, mood swings and ultimately diabetes, heart disease and cancer.

Remember Everything is within your control. You have to want to be well, and eat well, to feel fantastic.

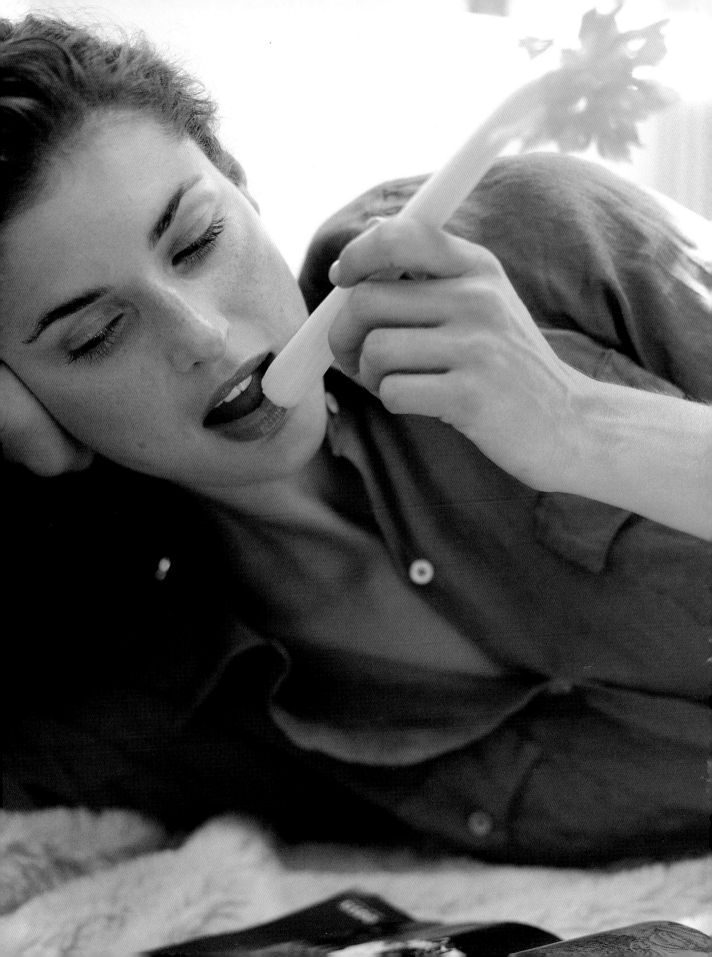

What you do in these 21 days

if you're 20-35

Trying out the latest diet is often 'a trend thing' in your early years, but this can lead to yo-yo dieting long-term. That's unhealthy for every part of your body, including your skin and your hair. Try this regime and see how good balanced eating patterns can make you feel.

● Avoid alcohol bingeing at parties. It severely depletes essential vitamins and minerals, encourages snacking, and sends your blood-sugar levels soaring.
● If you're busy on the run, keep vital healthy snacks such as nuts and seeds to hand in your bag.
● Make the effort to turn round your diet to include lots of the antioxidant vegetables that will keep your body and your skin looking better for longer.
● Slow something down in your life if you're feeling stressed. Even eating more slowly aids digestion and that helps you in the long run.

...or 35-50

Eating late (due to pressures of work and children), TV dinners, quick sugary energy snacks, all lead to malnutrition, though you may, in fact, have gained some weight. Cellulite may also now be more pronounced due to poor lymphatic drainage and increased amounts of toxins, resulting from your hectic lifestyle. Good nutrition and exercise can still turn things around.

● Focus. You'll especially benefit from the initial, more intensive detox to cleanse from the inside.
● Keep moving. Moderate exercise that works for you (see chapter 2) coupled with this 21-day eating plan achieves the best results – faster.
● Enjoy it. This isn't punishment – it's about finding the new you.
● Bump up your cellulite-busting regime (chapters 3 and 4): take in lots of body brushing and exfoliation. Massage problem areas with firming treatment creams and potions, and indulge in a few weekly detox treatments.

...or 50 and over

Excellent nutrition is one of the greatest anti-agers of all time for your face, body and inner health. By cutting substantial amounts of wheat and sugar out of your diet, you should feel as much of an improvement in your limbs as you see in your face.

● Up those vital antioxidant red, green, orange and yellow fruits and vegetables.
● Focus on fish. Once protein is reintroduced into your diet for supper on day 7, make the most of oily fish for its omega-3 oil, which is vital for cholesterol reduction, joints and an effective immune system.
● Drink lots of fluids – especially bottled water. It does the body so much more good inside and out than we know.

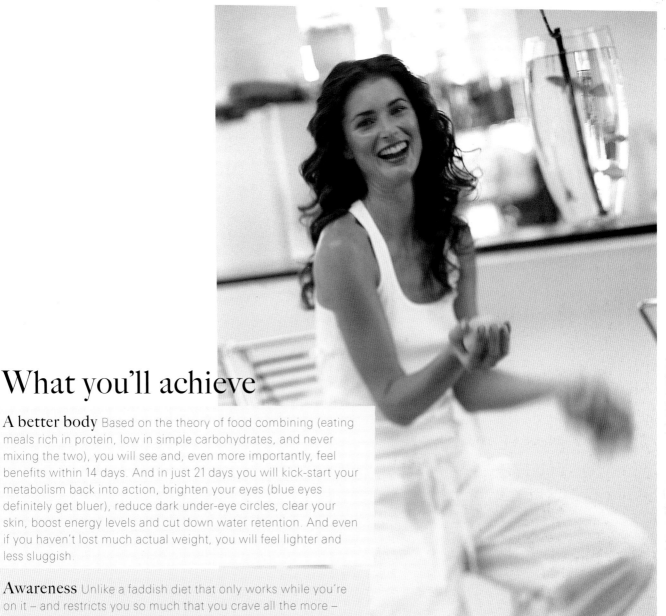

What you'll achieve

A better body Based on the theory of food combining (eating meals rich in protein, low in simple carbohydrates, and never mixing the two), you will see and, even more importantly, feel benefits within 14 days. And in just 21 days you will kick-start your metabolism back into action, brighten your eyes (blue eyes definitely get bluer), reduce dark under-eye circles, clear your skin, boost energy levels and cut down water retention. And even if you haven't lost much actual weight, you will feel lighter and less sluggish.

Awareness Unlike a faddish diet that only works while you're on it – and restricts you so much that you crave all the more – this programme will help you appreciate what you're eating and finally curb those sugar cravings. By following a better, more informed regime, you'll learn to listen to your body and become more aware of what it really needs. So, instead of succumbing thankfully to old eating habits when the programme ends, you'll have established new eating patterns – hopefully for life.

Knowledge Understanding nutrition will help you learn more about your health too. Why does it matter? Because food is life. And when we eat better, we feel better in ourselves, and our lives are the richer for it.

A better you Making an effort for you – be it cutting out sugar or alcohol – will have great repercussions. What better way could there be to convince yourself that you love your body than by taking better care of it from now on?

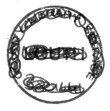

your nutrition kit

THESE CHECKLISTS COMPRISE THE ITEMS
MENTIONED IN THE 21-DAY NUTRITION
PROGRAMME MENUS. FEEL FREE TO BUY MORE
OF FEWER TYPES OF FRUIT AND SWAP WITH
SUGGESTIONS YOU MAY NOT LIKE - IT'S
YOUR PLAN TO TAILOR TO YOUR TASTEBUDS.
THE VARIETY IS THERE TO RELIEVE
BOREDOM, BUT CONVENIENCE MEANS DON'T
WASTE WHAT YOU'VE ALREADY BOUGHT.
THESE LISTS MAY ALSO BE A USEFUL
REMINDER, POST PLAN, OF YOUR BETTER-
EATING REGIME SO KEEP A COPY
BY YOU WHENEVER YOU GO SHOPPING

Salad stuff & vegetables

Asparagus, Avocado, Bean sprouts,
Broccoli, Carrots, Cauliflower, Celery,
Chicory, Courgettes, Cucumber, Endive,
Fennel, Green beans, Iceberg lettuce,
Lamb's lettuce, Mange-tout, Mushrooms,
Onions (shallots have great flavour & red
onions look great in salads), Peppers (red,
yellow, orange and green), Radish, Rocket,
Spinach, Sweetcorn, Tomatoes &
Watercress

Fruit

Apples, Bananas (not on days 3–7), Berries,
Cherries, Grapefruit, Grapes, Kiwi fruit,
Lemons, Limes, Mangoes, Melons,
Nectarines, Oranges, Papaya, Passion fruit,
Peaches, Pears, Pineapple, Plums,
Raspberries, Satsumas & Strawberries

Protein

Bacon, Cheese (feta or haloumi, goat's
cheese, mozzarella, parmesan), Chicken,
Eggs, Fish (salmon, sole, plaice &
monkfish), King prawns, Lamb, Milk, Nuts
(almonds are the lowest in fat and highest
in protein, brazil nuts, cashew nuts,
coconut, hazel nuts, pecans & walnuts),
Pulses (chick peas, red kidney beans,
lentils, & so on), Seeds (pumpkin, sesame &
sunflower) & Yoghurt (live natural)

Carbohydrate

Muesli, Potatoes (for baking), Rice cakes &
Wholegrains (brown rice, wholewheat
pasta & wholegrain bread, including rye
breads)

Drinks

Fruit and vegetable juices (for smoothies),
Fruit, herbal and green teas & Water

New rules

Food combining (originally devised by William Hay for the Hay diet) is based on the principle that mixing protein and carbohydrate in the same meal interferes with effective digestion.

Proteins are broken down in the stomach by acids, whereas carbs are broken down in the mouth, which is alkaline. And the two don't go. By separating the digestion of protein and carbohydrate, you reduce the demands made on your body and instantly start to relieve bloating, tiredness and that 'heavy' feeling.

And simple foods eaten raw or as near to their natural state as possible boost the metabolism, encourage weight loss and send your energy levels soaring. So there are just three basics to remember.

- Combine protein-rich foods (fish, meat, eggs, cheese, yoghurt, milk) with vegetables (any except potatoes) and pulses. This is the main stay of food combining: protein builds muscle and is more natural to our bodies than refined carbohydrates. And that's because historically we were meat-eaters and our bodies still process protein more naturally than the simple carbohydrates found in refined, processed foods.
- Combine complex carbohydrate-rich foods (potatoes, rice, wheat, oats, rye, pasta, bread) that give a slow release of energy with vegetables (as above) and sweet fruits (bananas, apples, coconut).
- Eat fast-fermenting fruits (berries, cherries, grapefruit, mango, oranges, papaya, peaches, pears, pineapple, plums) alone or half an hour before or after a meal.

Old eating habits

Egg on toast, meat and two veg (one being potato), ham salad sandwich, spaghetti bolognese

New alternatives

Egg and bacon, meat and three or four veg (all coloured green, red, orange, yellow – preferably no root vegetables), ham salad, spaghetti napoletana

portion control

Let yourself feel indulged without eating to excess. Consider a portion the equivalent of half a cup. With the exception of salads and vegetables, which you can eat in abundance, use this as your guide for foods such as nuts, fruit, brown rice and rice.

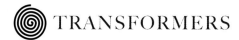
week
one

On days 1-2 you eat light, still quite filling meals, cutting out stimulants such as alcohol, coffee and sugar to prime your body for the more intense detox regime of days 3-7.

When do I start?
Cutting back hugely on your food intake may make you feel a little lethargic. So choose a time when you're not too stressed, say a long weekend. But the plan does provide you with enough to carry on working and exercising. In fact, you'll feel strangely euphoric come day 7. By day 14 this feeling should be replaced by amazing energy.

Eating to cleanse
During your intensive 5-day detox you will be cutting out wheat, dairy, caffeine and simple carbohydrates such as refined sugar to give your body an intensive cleanse. And to kick-start this whole cleansing process your body needs a rest from your usual eating pattern. So over the next seven days you'll be eating masses of fresh fruit and vegetables packed with essential nutrients, many of which may have been lacking in your diet.

Be creative with your food
You can create delicious and satisfying salads by mixing together lots of different ingredients. But make sure that you use masses of leafy green vegetables. And don't underestimate a salad leaf. All of them contain the pigment chlorophyll and that has the most amazing detoxifying properties to help revitalize your body and clear your system – FAST.

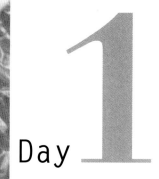

Day 1

Wake up
Cut 2–3 slices of lemon and squeeze them into a mug of hot water

Breakfast
Muesli with chopped strawberries

Energy treat
Raspberries

Lunch
Tomato, mozzarella and avocado salad with a green salad on the side

Supper
Chargrilled chicken kebabs
Grill or barbecue one chicken breast per person, with strips of red and green peppers, courgettes, mushrooms and baby tomatoes. (Use this time to cook an extra piece of chicken for tomorrow's lunch.) Once cooked, slice and cube, and then skewer together with the vegetables. Improvise: a stem of rosemary, stripped of leaves save for the first 10cm (4in) makes a great skewer.

Start the day The hot-water-and-lemon habit is cleansing and refreshing and gets your digestive juices going first thing.

Stock up on Fresh herbs for flavour: oregano, basil and tarragon are a few classic favourites that go wonderfully with salads.

Day 2

Wake up
Cut 2–3 slices of lemon and squeeze them into a mug of hot water

Breakfast
Mixed berries (strawberries, raspberries, blackberries and bilberries) and a spoonful of live natural yoghurt

Energy treat
Banana

Lunch
Chicken and avocado salad

Supper
Grilled salmon, steamed courgettes, green beans and mange-tout

The fastest salad around

spinach leaves
green salad leaves
½ avocado
200g (7oz) chicken, grilled
squeeze of lemon juice
fresh-ground pepper
olive oil (optional)

Sliced the grilled chicken. Place all the leaves together in a bowl; scatter the avocado on top, and then the chicken. Add a sprinkle of lemon juice and salt and a crackle of pepper to taste. Avoid salad dressing if possible – try just a drizzle of olive oil if you need something.

Day 3

Wake up
Fresh slices of lemon in a cup of hot water (add honey to taste if required)

Breakfast
Fresh fruit salad of kiwi and strawberries

Energy treat
Pineapple slices

Lunch
Large mixed salad. Be creative with different leaves, and add small slices of radish, red onion, celery, tomato – anything that will make you enjoy it more.

Supper
Stir-fried baby vegetables
Choose from baby carrots, sweetcorn, beans, mange-tout, asparagus and courgettes – lightly tossed in olive oil to preserve all the goodness.

Needing a snack? Make sure you have plenty of ready-prepared snacks – nuts, fresh fruit, rice cakes, and so on – to hand to prevent you from snacking on sugar. Fill a big tub with lots of different nuts and seeds for variety, and carry this around with you to stabilize sugar levels. But, of course, don't overdo it either – restrict yourself to 25–35g (1–1 ¼oz) a day. Remember that you can toast them or blanch them for a change.

Stick with it You will get headaches at some stage – often around day 3 or 4. Usually a result of cutting down on caffeine and other toxins in your diet, they won't last. If you feel headachy or nauseous, take 500mg of vitamin C three times a day. And drink 1–2 litres (1 ¾–3 ½ pt) of bottled water daily to dilute those toxins and help flush them out faster.

Day 4

Wake up
Cut 2–3 slices of lemon and squeeze them into a mug of hot water

Breakfast
Grapefruit slices and a pile of mixed berries

Energy treat
Peach

Lunch
Mixed leafy salad

Supper
Home-made green vegetable soup or freshly pre-packed organic soup
Take your pick from asparagus, broccoli, cabbage, dahl, pea, spinach or watercress. (Avoid tinned soups – they often have high sugar and salt content – and check pre-packs carefully.)

Day 5

Wake up
Cut 2–3 slices of lemon and squeeze them into a mug of hot water

Breakfast
Purifying fruit salad: apple, grapes, papaya, peach, pear, pineapple

Energy treat
Orange

Lunch
Large mixed leafy salad

Supper
Medley of steamed baby vegetables: carrots, courgettes, sweetcorn, mange-tout, asparagus, peas, and broccoli and cauliflower heads.
Add a small knob of butter to taste if required.

Why detox? Your body reflects your inner health. When overworked and overburdened, the liver's efficiency is reduced. As a result toxins accumulate in the blood. A proper detox – ideally for three weeks as in this programme – increases the consumption of foods that encourage the elimination of toxins, helping your lymph system, liver, kidneys, digestion and skin to work more efficiently. Citrus fruits (lemon, lime, grapefruit, orange) help fortify the liver and are rich in antioxidant vitamin C, one of nature's most potent detoxifiers. So wherever possible, bump up on these.

Eat for energy Try an orange: sport fanatics rave about the energizing effects of a single orange taken while they're in training.

Don't miss Pre-washed bags of salad are so handy, especially if you're following this plan on your own. However, fresh leaves last longer and lettuce retains more vitamins when left intact.

Day 6

Wake up
Cut 2–3 slices of lemon and squeeze them into a mug of hot water

Breakfast
Whole papaya and the juice of a lime

Energy treat
Pear

Lunch
Large mixed leafy salad

Supper
Homemade fresh vegetable soup
Try colourful carrot or tomato soup, both are rich in betacarotene.

Day 7

Wake up
Cut 2–3 slices of lemon and squeeze them into a mug of hot water

Breakfast
Pineapple slices with cherries and berries

Energy treat
Apple

Lunch
Mixed leafy salad

Supper
Grilled tuna steak and a heap of crunchy steamed green vegetables

Cleansing juices The most effective cleansers are apple, grape, grapefruit, mango, papaya, peach, pear, pineapple, carrot, beetroot, and watercress. A glass of freshly squeezed juice is great – and it's a good energy boost too so try it when you're flagging. Pure pressed juice from a carton is the next best thing.

If you are feeling stressed Make sure you have plenty of those ready prepared snacks to hand (see day 3). Bad eating habits are exactly that – habits. Every time you fill up at a petrol station and buy that same chocolate bar you are giving in to your habits. Be more aware about how food makes you feel.

Why all these salads? Zero calories, they get your digestive juices going and are compatible with everything you eat on this diet. So anytime you don't think you've eaten enough, have another salad.

EVERY DAY ● DRINK TWO LITRES (3 ½ PT) OF BOTTLED WATER TO FLUSH THE TOXINS OUT OF YOUR BODY FASTER ● EAT AT LEAST FIVE 'COLOURED' PORTIONS OF FRUIT AND VEGETABLES (SEE PAGE 34) ● CHEW SLOWLY AND CALMLY TO EASE DIGESTION

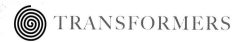

week one done

How do you feel?

Surprisingly light and bright? Or deprived? The whole detoxifying, cleansing thing is quite amazing, I think, because your entire body and mind feels energized and lighter... on less. If you aren't feeling this good, check you've been following the plan. No alcohol is a must. So is no coffee (just removing that from your life is regenerating) and no sugary snacks other than fruit.

● You should feel more balanced, refreshed and calm. Better nutrition highlights how you and your body feel. But don't let eating well be an obsession – you're just fuelling your body so it will work better.
● How easily have you been able to drink 2 litres (3 /pt) of water each day? If you're finding big bottles too daunting, decant into smaller bottles and congratulate yourself every time you finish one. Don't stress out about it. The fact that you're drinking any more will benefit your body.
● Re-assess yourself in the mirror. How do you look? Your skin tone may already have improved slightly. If not, wait till the end of next week.
● You should feel less sluggish. And flushing your kidneys means that you'll be urinating more often.
● Remember to treat your body with TLC, regularly exfoliating, massaging in lotions and potions, soaking with therapeutic essential oils. It's all in chapter 4. The more you treat your body with love, the more it will show.
● Keep your exercise going too (see chapter 2). You lose muscle if you lose weight and your body-fat percentage will go up unless you up your energy consumption through exercise and burn it all off.

Revisit these first seven days

whenever you want to look and feel better about yourself. But allow a month after the 21 days are up before you have another go at such an intense detox session.

If you have a young family

and find the menu hard to stick to, get them to join in. Add more protein for their portions, but avoid nuts where possible. They'll love the fruit salads in the morning and it's much better for them to eat wholefoods, if they will.

Need to shift a few pounds?

For those who've failed at weight-loss or reached a plateau, and are unable to shift any more, food combining can be a healthy, life-long eating regime.

keeping going

Learning to understand your body and how it works, its strengths and its weaknesses, is one of the best ways to boost your confidence. Self-image is always a complex issue, with both negative and positive attitudes developed from infancy through personal experiences that may run deep. That's why it is so important to be aware of the vital mind/body link through every part of this 21-day plan.

Record your feelings

Keep a notebook to write down how you feel after each meal. Eating a more nutritious diet needn't stop after these 21 days, and I'm hoping you'll want to continue. By recording how you feel, you'll become more aware of your body's response to foods. And while eating a more cleansing diet, any foods that trouble or have troubled you in the past may well be highlighted.

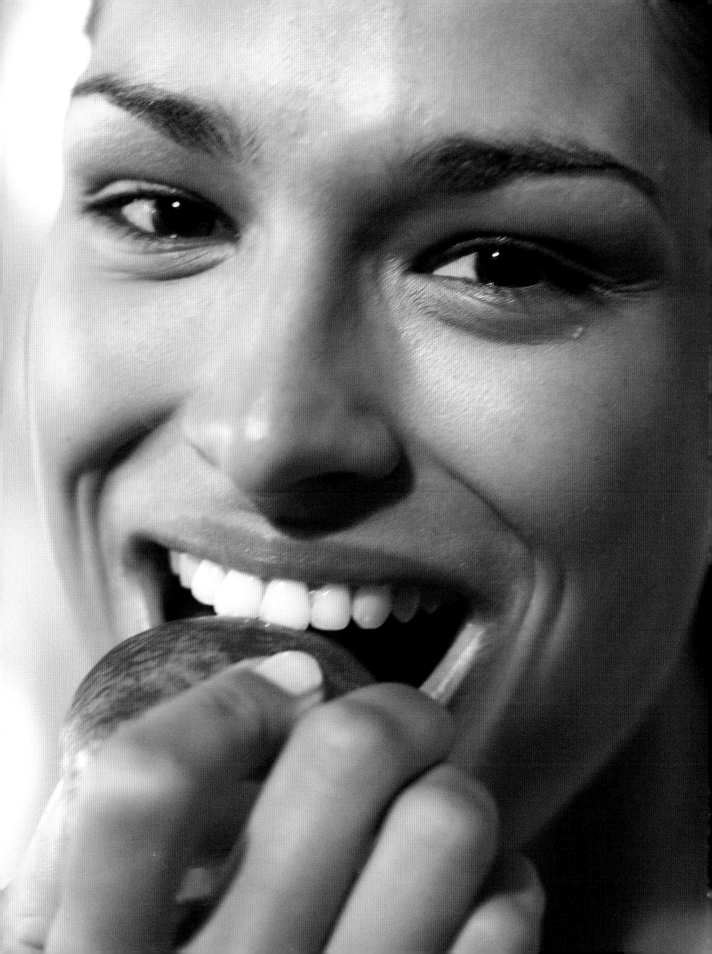

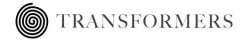

week
two

Well, that was the hard part. Now you'll be using the basic principles of food combining. Days 8–14 the menu is still light but more satisfying as you add in extra protein or a little carbohydrate to return you to a more 'normal' eating pattern.

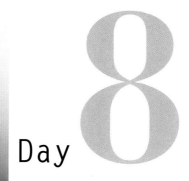

Day 8

Wake up
Herbal tea

Breakfast
Everyday fruit salad: apple, grapes, peach, pear and satsuma

Energy treat
Raspberries or make yourself a smoothie

Lunch
Mixed leafy salad with extra pulses: chick peas, haricot and kidney beans

Supper
One baked potato, a little butter and as much salad as you like

Lacking energy? Specific supplements can prove useful.

The B vitamins work together to produce energy, and are effective stress-beaters. Take as a vitamin-B complex. Natural sources: oily fish, wholegrains, pulses, green vegetables, mushrooms and eggs.

Co-enzyme Q10 is a natural substance that helps the body convert food into energy, but illness and ageing deplete it. Natural sources: oily fish, sesame seeds, peanuts and soya oil.

Iron is used to produce haemoglobin, which distributes oxygen in our blood. Low haemoglobin levels (anaemia) bring tiredness and an inability to exercise. But don't take a supplement without being tested: high doses of iron have been associated with a greater risk of heart disease. Natural sources: red meat, oatmeal, prunes, nuts and seeds, pulses and dried fruit. Minerals such as zinc, magnesium and chromium are also important energy nutrients, so think about taking a quality multi-mineral supplement.

Herbs can be useful too. Choose stimulating herbs that help to boost circulation and refresh the system during the regime. Rhodiola and ginseng are both useful for fatigue and stress.

Ruby smoothie

3 fresh peaches
1 banana
10 raspberries
2 tsp lemon juice
200ml (7fl oz) live natural yoghurt
honey (optional)

Chop all the fruit into a blender, adding the lemon juice. Blend for 15–20 seconds. Spoon in the yoghurt and blend again until smooth. Add honey to taste if needed

Day 9

Wake up
Herbal tea

Breakfast
Live natural yoghurt and a selection of fresh berries

Energy treat
Kiwi fruit

Lunch
Avocado and spinach salad

Supper
Vegetable paella

Veggie paella for two or three

3 peppers (red, green and yellow), sliced
2 shallots, sliced
4 tomatoes, skinned and sliced
3 tbsp olive oil
250g (8 ½oz) brown rice
small pinch saffron
300ml (½pt) light vegetable stock
1 tbsp thyme
1 garlic clove, chopped
seasoning

Preheat the oven to 180°C (350°F, Gas Mark 4). Heat the oil in a large flameproof dish. Add the shallots and cook until beginning to brown. Stir in the rice, a sprinkle of saffron and the stock, and bring to the boil. Mix in the rest of the vegetables, add the garlic, thyme and season.

Cover and bake in the oven for about 30 minutes. Keep an eye on it, and serve when all the liquid is absorbed and the rice tender.

Day 10

Wake up
Herbal tea

Breakfast
Muesli with semi-skimmed or skimmed milk, topped with fresh berries

Energy treat
Strawberries

Lunch
Large leafy egg salad

Supper
Tomato and lentil soup

Feeling sweet enough?
A sweet tooth is usually a habit picked up in childhood – often the result of treats or rewards. That's why, though your inclination is toward something sweet, you really can **turn it around**. But it takes determination and the full 21 days.

It's important to keep sugar levels in check, for not only does it affect your weight, it affects your mood too. The initial high you get from sweet foods (including bread) is quickly followed by tiredness, and irritability leads to low self-esteem. So eating comfort foods when you're low is the worst thing you can do as it causes blood-sugar levels to rise too quickly – only to fall even more.

● Stick to healthy snacks (see day 3).
● Don't skip breakfast.
● Eat small, well-balanced meals through the day. And you'll discover new energy levels and learn to handle stress.

Day 11

Wake up
Herbal tea

Breakfast
Grapefruit with blackberries (or other berries)

Energy treat
Pineapple

Lunch
Caesar salad

Supper
Roasted vegetables and couscous
If you've any leftover, keep to go with your salad for lunch tomorrow – day 12. The best vegetables for roasting are shallots, courgettes, mushrooms, peppers and tomatoes. Slice them all, place in an oven baking tray, drizzle with olive oil and sprinkle with a selection of mixed herbs. Roast for 10–15 minutes – check often so they don't burn. Serve with a leafy salad and shavings of parmesan.

Don't be clumsy with salads
Take time to prepare your food with care. Slice finely. A forkful of flavours – cucumber, tomato, avocado, pepper, celery and strips of lettuce – is much more appetising than great chunks.

Day 12

Wake up
Herbal tea

Breakfast
Fruit salad of pineapple, orange and grapefruit. Feel free to add any other fruit you like

Energy treat
Mango

Lunch
Mixed bean salad
Try the deli counter at your supermarket for a ready-made version if you're at work or busy.

Supper
Grilled sole/plaice/monkfish with steamed vegetables
Sprinkle the fish with lemon juice for extra flavour and serve with French beans, asparagus tips and strips of yellow and green courgettes.

Up your intake of sunflower, pumpkin or sesame seeds, especially if you feel run down or are overworked. Snack on them or add to salads.

REMEMBER TO ● KEEP MUNCHING HEALTHY SNACKS WHEN YOU NEED A PICK-ME-UP AND IT'S AGES TILL YOUR NEXT MEAL ● DRINK UP THAT BOTTLED MINERAL WATER ● EAT LITTLE AND OFTEN TO MAINTAIN BLOOD-SUGAR LEVELS

Day 13

Wake up
Herbal tea

Breakfast
Live natural yoghurt with nectarine or peaches (honey optional)

Energy treat
Apple

Lunch
Greek salad: cucumber, tomato, onion, and feta or haloumi cheese

Supper
Red pesto pasta with cherry tomatoes in basil and oregano
To make the tomatoes totally divine and add a fresh taste, cook the baby toms (10–12 for one) in a little olive oil and a sprinkle of oregano on a low heat until they are deliciously soft and their skins split. Pour over the cooked, drained pasta and stir in a helping of red pesto sauce. Sprinkle with freshly cut basil leaves.

Cutting down on stress Your body loses reserves of vitamin B, C and zinc when the pressure is on. But this regime boosts your daily intake of 'coloured' vegetables, wholegrains, nuts and fresh fruit, so you are now beginning to feel calmer from within.

Add honey to your yoghurt for a more natural sweet flavour if you really feel that you need it. But it encourages that sweet tooth so see if you can go without.

Day 14

Wake up
Herbal tea

Breakfast
Papaya and freshly squeezed lime

Energy treat
Pear (or a fresh fruit smoothie)

Lunch
Salad niçoise: tuna (this can be tinned for convenience), lettuce, boiled egg, tomato and black olives

Supper
Chicken and vegetable stir-fry

Fresh fruit smoothies are full of vital vitamins and so easy to make. If you love them, and prefer them to pieces of fruit, make up a whole batch for breakfast or keep it for your daily treat, or whenever you're tempted to sneak in a quick espresso. Try these flavours.

Mango, raspberry and banana
1 mango, 10–15 raspberries and 1 banana

Grapefruit, apple and mango
1 grapefruit, 2 apples and 1 mango

Pineapple, apricot and mango
Half a pineapple, 3 apricots and 1 mango

Make up according to the instructions on day 8. Don't forget to include the lemon and yoghurt.

week two over

How are you doing?

⚫ You should feel really alive and energized now. You're high on energy! You wake easily and feel fresh, and you aren't so tired in the evenings. And you're even able to stay awake on the sofa beyond 9pm. Pat yourself on the back. You're doing well.

⚫ Your digestive system should be working more effectively, with more regular bowel movements. These may be quite loose at times and this is natural. It's the result of your increased intake of fibre and your body is cleansing itself of all waste.

⚫ You're definitely looking good too. Your eyes are brighter, your skin is positively glowing all over with good health.

⚫ Your body feels leaner and lighter – you may not weigh much less but you feel so different.

⚫ Any water retention has vastly improved, though you need to keep drinking the water to boost the effect. Next week will be even better.

⚫ Depending on your personality, you're feeling wonderful surges of happiness (euphoria about nothing at all) or calm (focused, no-hassle-it-won't-bother-me) and peaceful.

⚫ Keep going. If it's summer, alcohol could be really tempting. Make yourself some exotic smoothies, and add lemon and lime to glasses of chilled water or cleansing juices.

⚫ Keep pampering your body. Now that you're seeing results, really get into body brushing (see chapter 4) and boost that progress.

⚫ Hopefully you've got the exercise bug by this stage. Your efforts will only ever achieve good results.

from the inside out

Antioxidants One reason why fruit and veg are so good for you is that they are packed with antioxidants. Oxidization happens when harmful cells (or free radicals) destroy your body's cells. Produced as the body burns oxygen, and as a result of too much sunlight, smoking, pollution and other environmental chemicals, free radicals cause the body and mind to age, and trigger life-threatening diseases. Antioxidants are the chemicals that disarm free radicals.

The best-known antioxidants include vitamins C and E and betacarotene, but there has been a lot of research on the protective effects of powerful but lesser known antioxidants, such as lycopene and bioflavinoids. Red, orange, yellow and green foods are the best source of anti-ageing antioxidants. If you eat a healthy diet rich in them, you shouldn't need to supplement, especially betacarotene which can be toxic in excess. Just listen to your body. When it is in balance, you simply radiate health and vitality.

Water Up to 70 per cent of your body is water, so you need a plentiful supply just to function normally. As soon as your fluid levels drop, your body processes slow down, bringing headaches, fatigue, aching joints and dry skin. Dehydration also makes you more vulnerable to urinary infections, high blood pressure, indigestion and constipation. In addition, your immune system will function less effectively. And you may put on weight. That's why you need to make sure you get enough, so aim for that 2 litres (3 ½pt) a day target, remembering that mineral water is free from the chemicals found in tap water. And when your exercise plan really gets going, you'll need to increase this amount because you'll be losing more water through perspiration.

maximize your superfoods

Avocados are everywhere in this plan. That's because they contain more energy and nutrients than any other fruit. Packed with folic acid, vitamins A, B6 and C, potassium and protein, they are almost a complete food.

● Avocados are brain food. They are high in lecithin, which helps to improve mental abilities and memory.

● They're great for your skin because they contain EFAs (essential fatty acids). The best fat you can consume, they 'oil' your skin from inside, smoothing and softening.

● They're high in lutein, a powerful antioxidant which is known to protect against eye diseases such as cataracts and may protect skin from sun damage.

Oily fish is extremely high in omega-3 oil, which has many benefits and is high in EFAs. For example, it is known to protect against heart disease, blood clotting and arthritis. Western diets are rich in omega-6, but very low in omega-3.

● Oily fish can reduce chances of a second heart attack by 30 per cent. Salmon, mackerel, sardines and anchovies have the highest omega-3. (Only tuna does not retain omega fats after canning.)

● Oily fish protects against inflammatory conditions such as rheumatoid arthritis and psoriasis.

● Oily fish cheers you up – it's true! Researchers found that countries with high oily-fish consumption have less depression.

Broccoli is packed full of goodness. It is high in vitamin A and has more vitamin C than oranges.

● Broccoli is rich in folic acid, a vital B group vitamin. And recent research shows that folic acid lowers the levels of a type of cholesterol called homocysteine – too much in the bloodstream is believed to be the first step to clogged arteries.

● Broccoli contains phytochemicals that help switch off cancer-causing substances. They also kill off the bacterium *Helicobacter pylori*, which is thought to cause most stomach ulcers.

● It's high in sulphur, which detoxifies the blood and keeps skin and hair healthy; iron, which helps bring energy to every cell in the body; and chlorophyll, a blood purifier.

Strawberries and raspberries contain vitamins B, C and E and high levels of iron, calcium, and silica, all essential for cell growth.

● A single punnet of either delivers a high dose of the antioxidants that help prevent heart disease.

● Raspberries have a gently detoxifying effect on the body.

● Both berries are high in folic acid (see broccoli, left).

● Strawberries and raspberries are rich in ellagic acid, which is believed to help protect against cancer.

Tomatoes are rich in vitamins and folic acid.

● They have significant amounts of the powerful antioxidant lycopene, which has been shown to lower the risk of prostate cancer, and it's believed to reduce the risk of other cancers too. But to get the benefits you need to eat cooked tomatoes because heat breaks down the cell walls and that's what releases lycopene for absorption by the body.

● Tomatoes contain the flavinoid rutin, which helps to strengthen the capillaries of the bloodstream.

● Tomatoes are a good source of vitamins A and C, as well as calcium and phosphorus, which together build bone, and potassium, which lowers blood pressure.

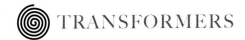

week
three

Day 15

Socialize. Invite people round for supper again – the menu's just become much more interesting. Keep them busy with lots of delicious nuts, while you prepare a supper that starts with a green salad or green vegetable soup. Follow that with a main course from the plan. (The more colour you add, the more impressive it looks so perhaps opt for something with peppers.) Then serve an exotic fruit salad with mango, papaya, passion fruit and kiwi over half an hour later. Dandelion coffee is caffeine free and a healthier alternative.

Wake up
Herbal tea

Breakfast
Muesli with semi-skimmed or skimmed milk and topped with strawberries and raspberries

Energy treat
Raspberries

Lunch
Veggie rice salad
Chop the reserved roasted vegetables from the previous night finely and mix with brown rice. If you prepare it the night before, you can save time today. Pack and take to work or on a picnic.

Supper
Lamb kebabs
Either oven grill or barbecue. Slice courgettes (yellow and green) and peppers, and once cooked wrap one or two different slices around each chunk of lamb. Intersperse with shallots, tomatoes and mushrooms.

Cleanse yourself naturally
Drinking masses of mineral water will encourage your kidneys to flush away toxins. But the easy passage of food through the intestine is also vital for the cleansing process. Increasing your intake of roughage with the leaves, stalks and roots of vegetables, as well as the skins and seeds of fruit, helps considerably.

Day 16

Wake up
Herbal tea

Breakfast
Fruit kebabs of kiwi, melon, pineapple, peach, pear and strawberries. Or whatever else you have to hand.

Energy treat
Papaya and freshly squeezed lime

Lunch
An open sandwich (i.e. one slice of wholemeal bread) topped with rocket, vine tomatoes and balsamic vinegar

Supper
Warm smoked chicken, bacon, spinach and avocado salad
It takes no time at all and tastes delicious – almost too good to be good.

Don't skimp Avocados have a reputation for being very high in fat, so weight-conscious people often avoid them. However, like nuts, the fat avocados contain is mono-unsaturated, and has been shown to lower artery-clogging 'bad' cholesterol, making it a great defence against heart disease and strokes.

Missing that espresso? It takes at least a week to wean yourself off the effects of caffeine, but it has a huge effect on your energy levels. Try green tea, a natural antioxidant that boosts the immune system, prevents tooth decay and inhibits cancer.

Curb your cravings If you truly, hand-on-heart stick to this 21-day regime, you will find at the end that your desire for all things sweet and starchy has gone. And with it your need to stabilize your blood-sugar levels.

You're cutting out all those refined, sugary and starchy foods – including white bread, white rice, white pasta – that quickly release sugar into your bloodstream. And you're replacing them with foods that release sugar more slowly: wholegrain foods, pulses, fresh fruit and vegetables.

Small meals throughout the day also help to avoid slumps in blood sugar. After large meals, your blood-sugar levels can rise dramatically. In response, your body secretes insulin to help bring the levels back to normal. Cells use insulin to turn sugar into energy, but too much insulin can cause sugar to be turned into body fat. The solution is to keep to your food-combining principles and exercise more if you can.

Salad sandwiches are a convenient way to cope when you're at work, and they still comply with food-combining principles. But not every day. Compensate for the wholegrain bread with lots of leaves, tomatoes, cucumber, and so on. And cucumber sandwiches on their own are allowed too – but make sure there's extra cucumber inside so the ratio of vegetable to bread is greater (and season with black pepper rather than salt).

REMEMBER TO ● RELISH EVERY MOUTHFUL WHILE CHEWING CONSIDERATELY ● CURB HUNGER PANGS WITH RICE CAKES AND A GLASS OF WATER

Day 17

Wake up
Herbal tea

Breakfast
One slice of wholegrain toast and a tiny dab of butter, or with honey if desired (and no butter)

Energy treat
Pineapple

Lunch
Mixed bean and pasta salad

Supper
Roasted red peppers stuffed with vegetable rice and served with a leafy salad

Day 18

Wake up
Herbal tea

Breakfast
Fruit salad of melon, mango, passion fruit, kiwi and strawberries

Energy treat
Melon

Lunch
Improvise with strips of egg, bacon and chicken, tossed together with some salad leaves for a protein-rich, deliciously easy but impressive salad

Supper
Dahl soup

Dahl soup

400g (14oz) dried chick peas
    (soaked overnight)
4–5 shallots
6 garlic cloves
pepper (avoid salt if you can)
5 tbsp olive oil
3–4 tsp cumin seeds
750ml (1 ¼pt) vegetable stock
juice of ½ lemon
fresh mint

Drain the chick peas and cover with about 4cm (1 ½in) of water. Add 2 shallots and 3 garlic cloves, all whole. Boil for 5 minutes, then lower the heat and simmer for 1 hour until tender, adding pepper (and salt).

Meanwhile chop the remaining shallots and garlic and soften in another pan, using half the oil and 2 tsp cumin (freshly ground). Then add half the stock and set aside until needed.

When the chick peas are cooked, discard the shallots and garlic. Add the contents of the other pan and the lemon juice to the chick peas and stir. Blend half the mixture until smooth and pour into a large saucepan. Blend the rest of the mixture lightly, leaving a little texture.

Combine both halves, add the remaining stock, and heat for 10 minutes. Garnish with mint and a sprinkle of cumin seeds.

Day 19

Wake up
Herbal tea

Breakfast
Muesli with semi-skimmed or skimmed milk. Add plenty of chopped hazel nuts, blanched almonds and cashew nuts and some delicious fruit.

Energy treat
Pear

Lunch
Warm goat's cheese and mixed leaf salad

Supper
Poached salmon and lightly buttered, steamed vegetables of your choice

Better cooking To maintain the nutritional content of your food, steam, poach, bake, grill or stir-fry, and avoid re-heating which further depletes essential nutrients. It honestly tastes better too.

Supplements? Bump up all the good work you've been doing to ensure that your body gets everything it needs right now. Take a multi-vitamin and one capsule of evening primrose oil or omega-3 oil with a full glass of water at meal times.

Day 20

Wake up
Herbal tea

Breakfast
Fruit kebabs of kiwi, melon, pineapple, mango and strawberries. Or whatever you have to hand.

Energy treat
Mango

Lunch
Pasta napoletana
Make tomato sauce more exciting with the addition of red peppers and fresh herbs.

Supper
Lemon chicken with steamed vegetables (the choice is yours)
When cooking a whole chicken, wash the bird, slice a couple of lemons in half and stuff them inside. Wrap in foil and cook as usual. The meat is just spiked with lemon, giving a wonderfully refreshing twist to the flavour.

Avoid buying tempting snacks Keep to the outer aisles at the supermarket. This is where they tend to keep the healthy basics – fresh fish, meat, eggs, fruit and vegetables. Order on line, or get someone else to do the shopping!

Eat a handful of nuts before each meal A small amount of healthy fat slows down digestion, making your stomach feel full for longer. So, eaten before a meal, nuts can persuade you to eat less. Healthy fats are also derived from fish, olive oil and avocado. Rich in mono- or polyunsaturated fats, they keep your blood sugar more stable and help your body absorb fat-soluble vitamins A, D, E and K.

Day 21

Wake up
Herbal tea

Breakfast
Wholegrain toast with a smear of honey or jam

Energy treat
Banana

Lunch
Lemon chicken and avocado salad
Use some of the chicken from supper on day 20

Supper
King prawn kebabs with peppers, onions, mushrooms and courgettes

---

Skin essentials By now you should have noticed a real improvement in your skin. Increasing your intake of multi-coloured fruit and vegetables, and oily fish, also ups your intake of these vital nutrients.

vitamin B complex repairs
vitamin C boosts collagen production
vitamin E anti-ageing and balancing
betacarotene converts into vitamin A and that's essential for cell renewal
EFAs these essential fatty acids play a vital part in softening and smoothing skin texture

how
did you do?

You've finished. Great. How do you feel? How do you look? It wasn't that hard, was it? What bits did you enjoy? Which bits were the hardest? Did you stick to everything? Did you record it all so you can remember? Do you understand what makes your body healthy? How has it changed your attitude to food? Does it taste better? Could you food combine for life? If not, why not? You're going to do the programme again, aren't you? Not tomorrow, but maybe in a month or three. Turn to page 238 for programmes to try any time.

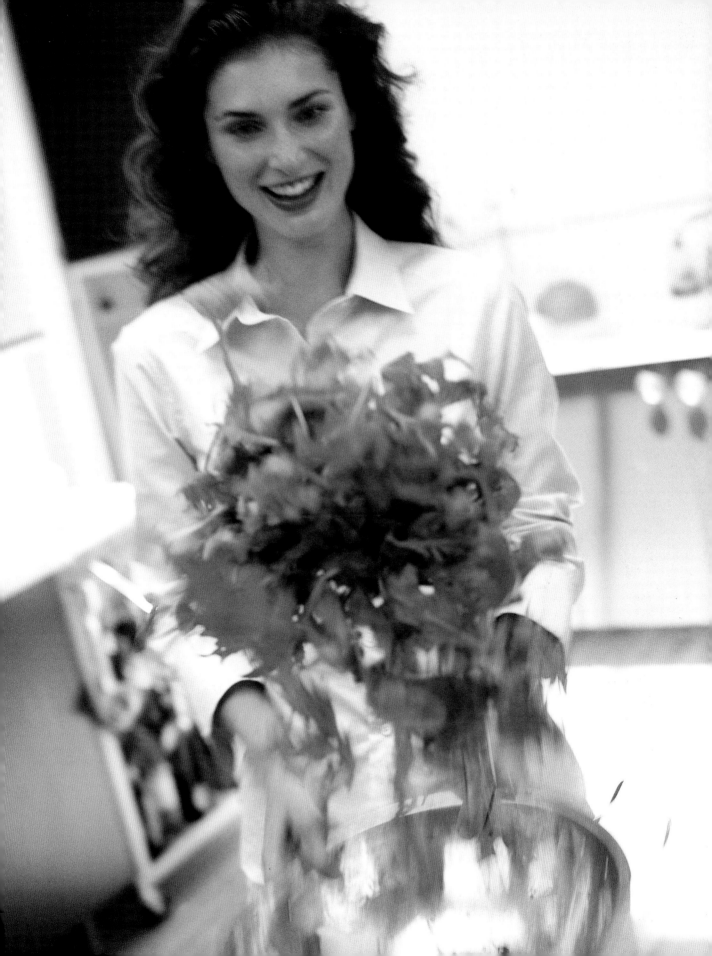

Leave out the teabag Every time you 'make the tea', stop at the hot water and leave out the caffeine. Drinking hot water is surprisingly refreshing and Chinese medicine values hot water over a glass of icy cold water because it's less of a shock to your system.

Keep drinking that water You've heard it all before, but water is vital for all your body's functions. Don't wait until you're thirsty – aim for 2 litres (3 ½pt) taken through the day, and not all at once, or you'll just overload your kidneys. If you're dehydrated, you're circulating less oxygen round the body, so you naturally feel more sluggish.

Suffering from bad breath? It's all those toxins you're shedding. Take vitamin C and calcium supplements, chew on a bit of parsley, bump up your intake of live yoghurt and drink peppermint tea.

Think positive, think tasty You and your mind can make all the difference with this regime. Focus on the words 'delicious', 'refreshing', 'tasty' rather than the words 'diet', 'restricted' or 'boring'. Success for life is all in the mind.

Body shaping for the beach Limit your sugary, processed carbohydrates even more. Lose the rice and potatoes that bloat your stomach.

Often tired or lethargic? You may lack essential group B vitamins or magnesium and iron. Try eating several low-fat snacks through the day, and avoid quick boosters such as caffeine or sweets, which only exacerbate fatigue over time.

fast track

Cook in volume A whole chicken will cover your meals for three days if you're following this plan alone. If you have a family, incorporate their meals with yours.

Eat peanuts! They are a good source of mono-unsaturated fatty acids, magnesium and folate (folic acid), vitamin E, copper, arginine and fibre, according to research. Although peanuts are often avoided because they are thought to be high in fat, they are actually rich in the types of fats that reduce the risk of cardiovascular disease.

Choose your tomatoes Tomato contains high amounts of the antioxidant lycopene, which is known to help prevent prostate cancer, but is believed to help prevent ovarian and breast cancer too. Tomatoes that have been bred, grown and picked for maximum lycopene content are slightly pear shaped and bantam-egg sized, and, most importantly, they are red the whole way through, not green or fawn.

Make some for lunch too Supper meals such as roast vegetables and couscous (day 11) or veggie paella (day 9) can be eaten cold the next day for lunch with a salad to save money and time. All the recipes are interchangeable after the first detox week. The most important thing is to follow the rules of food combining (see page 23).

Take five or more pieces of fruit and vegetables (approximately 450g/1lb) each day. Ideally half the food you eat should be fresh fruits and raw vegetables.

Salad for guests Rocket, sun-blushed tomatoes and shavings of parmesan with a drizzle of balsamic vinegar and cracked pepper. Very delicious – and a great salad if you're entertaining on this regime. Add a little Parma ham to glam it up (but not for you on days 3–7).

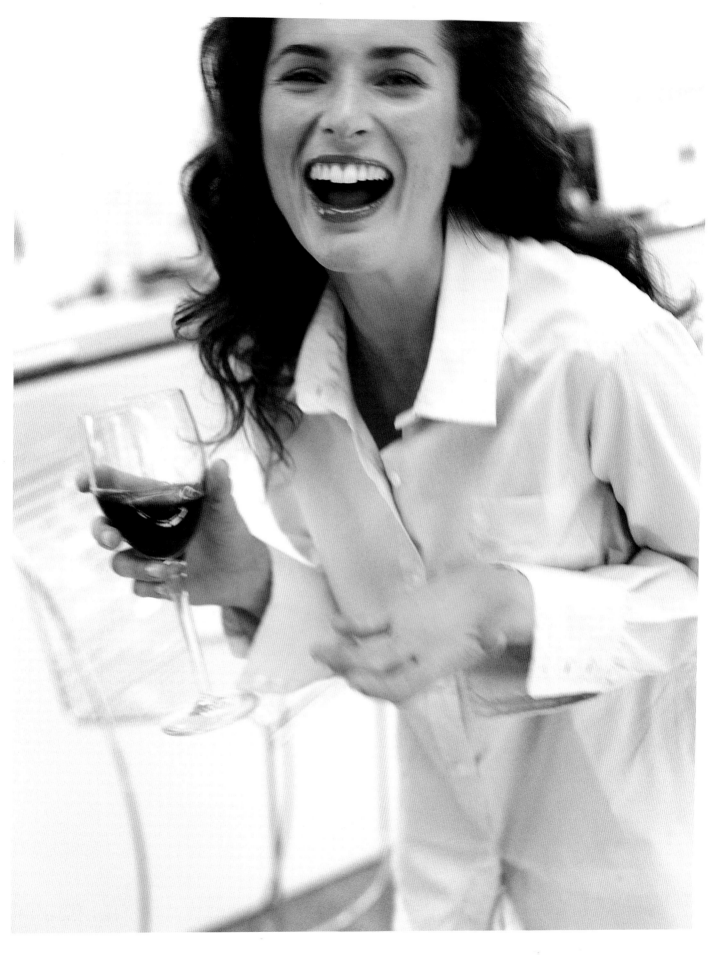

keeping it going

Don't treat yourself with food

Buy a pretty dress, see a show, have a massage. There are far nicer, better ways to indulge yourself.

Seek balance

● Keep plenty of healthy snacks and fresh fruit at hand. You'll be less likely to succumb to temptation.

● Make yourself a weekly food plan. Use weeks two and three from the programme to plan a week's menus of meals that you adore. Copy page 22 and keep it with you whenever you're grocery shopping. It will help – less wasted food and fewer temptations – and it keeps you on track.

● While you're inspired, search through all your cookbooks for recipes that can be enjoyed while food combining. Add some of these to your plan. Change it every two to four weeks. But, most importantly, plan ahead.

● Order by internet – you'll be less tempted to make impulse buys based on the aroma and packaging.

● Cut back on sugar in the household. Treats should be treats. When they become a regular part of your diet or that of your family and children, it's time to re-assess and restart the programme. If you think children need sugary foods, think again. Alongside tooth decay, many of today's childhood behavioural problems are believed to stem from a poor diet. 'Treat' children with an afternoon somewhere special, a comic, a story, more of your time…anything but sugar.

● Every three months do the first seven days of the programme again. A cleansing of the palate promotes healthier eating and a healthier lifestyle.

Focus on the new you. After all, you now...

● Always eat breakfast. Studies show that a good breakfast significantly enhances mental performance and improves memory during the day. Choose porridge, muesli, an egg or fruit rather than a sugar-laden, pre-packed cereal.

● Never skip lunch. Low blood sugar slows your ability to process information and reduces attention span.

● Drink natural teas or water. Don't use coffee or sugary food to keep you going when you're stressed. Try nibbling on fruit.

● Boost your vitamin C intake. High vitamin C levels are associated with improved mood, intelligence and memory. Snack on satsumas or take a supplement each morning.

Choose a better path

The best way to keep it going – because you really can – is to follow all the principles of the eating plan for life. Or, if not for life, maybe for the weekdays – and then relax a little at the weekends. Surely now you've seen and felt the results you don't want to revert to your old ways?

● Cut back on alcohol. Now and then have a glass of red wine. In moderation wine can actually benefit your health: the grapes contain powerful antioxidants called procyanadins, which protect the body from the inside out. But too much and you'll be back into your blood-sugar imbalance before you can say 'boo'.

● Increase the amount of 'coloured' fruit and vegetables you eat forever. Remember that minimum of 450g (1lb) of fruit and vegetables a day (that's five apple-sized portions). And ideally, half the foods you eat should be fresh fruits and raw vegetables: consumed in their natural state, they are rich in anti-ageing antioxidants. Limit the amount of meat and fish to a total of four meals a week – at lunch and supper. There is considerable evidence that this regime significantly reduces the risk of heart disease, stroke and some cancers. And recent Canadian research found that eating more vegetables and soya-based products could be as effective at reducing cholesterol as statins, the drugs that have been used to treat high cholesterol levels for 15 years.

● Maintain the nutritional content of cooked food as much as possible by steaming, poaching, baking or stir-frying, and avoid re-heating, which further depletes essential nutrients.

● Avoid margarine, fried foots and sugar (see page 111).

● Cut down on caffeine, which inhibits the absorption of vitamins and minerals. Experiment with herbal (flower, fruit and green) teas, and occasional cups of hot water with or without the lemon. (Too many lemon drinks after the 21-day programme is over and your dentist won't approve because citric acid attacks the enamel.)

● Drink 2 litres (3 /pt) water every single day.

Better digestion

● Don't eat immediately after work. Relax and de-stress first.

● Don't eat when angry or upset.

● Don't eat quickly. Take the time to eat properly. Chewing your food slowly has been found to help relieve stress.

● Don't eat a large meal just before you prepare for bed.

● Don't drink as you eat. It dilutes digestive enzymes.

● Sit upright and focus on your food.

● Eat small meals and snacks. Don't go more than two and a half hours without eating, and always eat that big breakfast. And remember: better digestion goes hand in hand with relaxation. Find yourself at least 10 minutes of calm every day. Whatever you choose, make it something that works for you, so you will constantly turn to it in stressful situations.

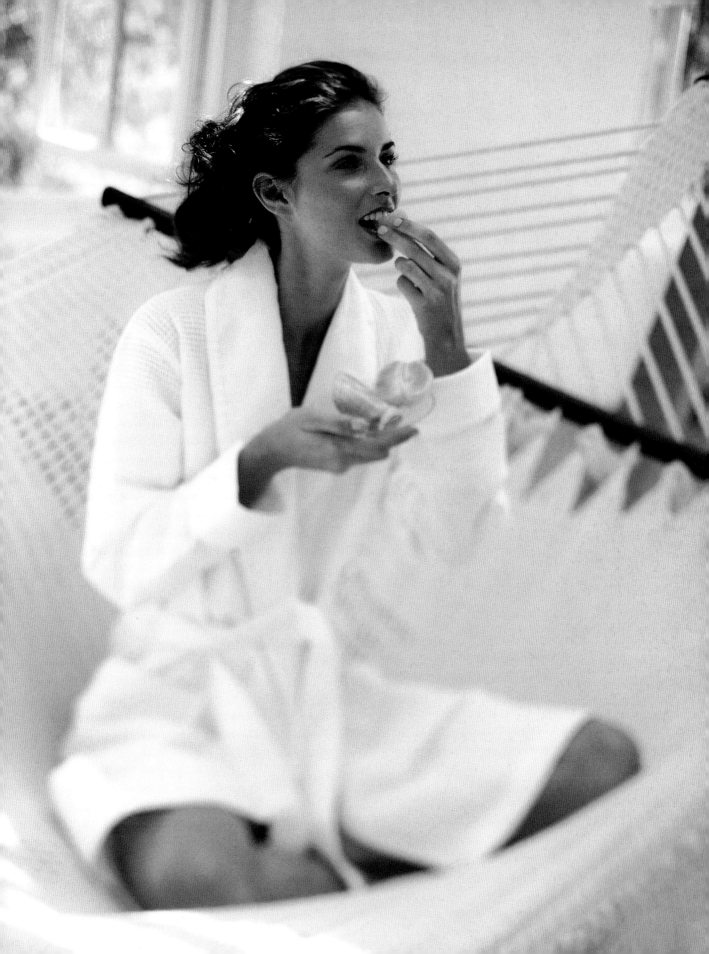

21 DAYS

TO A

FITTER

HEALTHIER

BODY

Nothing makes you feel so complete in yourself as moving and breathing in harmony through exercise. Time to take action and let your body take shape.

Your fitness programme

This fitness programme is designed to suit you and your lifestyle. I'm not asking you to go to a gym unless you do already. The aim is simply to start you exercising a little more, whatever your current fitness level. The daily regime is based on a series of gentle to moderate 20-minute exercise routines that are achievable by beginners, brief enough to keep you wanting to do them, and beneficial whatever your age.

BOREDOM IS THE NO. 1 REASON WHY PEOPLE GIVE UP ON EXERCISE. VARY YOUR REGIME AND YOU'LL STICK TO IT.

What do I do? Each day you exercise in three quite separate ways, using gentle yoga stretches, easy-to-achieve aerobics (probably fast-paced walking), and spot-toning exercises based on pilates that can be done at home. It's a routine that's easy to remember, not too repetitive and it can be adapted to fit in with your day. Combined with great nutrition and an active skincare and bodycare regime, you really will make dramatic improvements in your sense of wellbeing.

Why 20 minutes? Well, everyone can manage that, can't they? And that's the time it takes during aerobic workouts such as walking for your body to start burning fat – anything less won't do it. So in weeks two and three you can, if you wish, increase your aerobic exercise and be confident that you're working at a pace that will efficiently burn off fat.

I just don't have the time Your Fitness programme has been designed to fit in with your day – every day – but don't feel that you have to do it all. Getting a balance that works for you is the most important thing. Bear in mind that 30 minutes exercise a day, five times a week, is now said to be the minimum to keep your body fit and healthy. So just set yourself realistic goals using your daily planner, and you will feel triumphant rather than despondent. If you only get to do 10 minutes at each session, well it's better than 5, and ten times better than nothing at all.

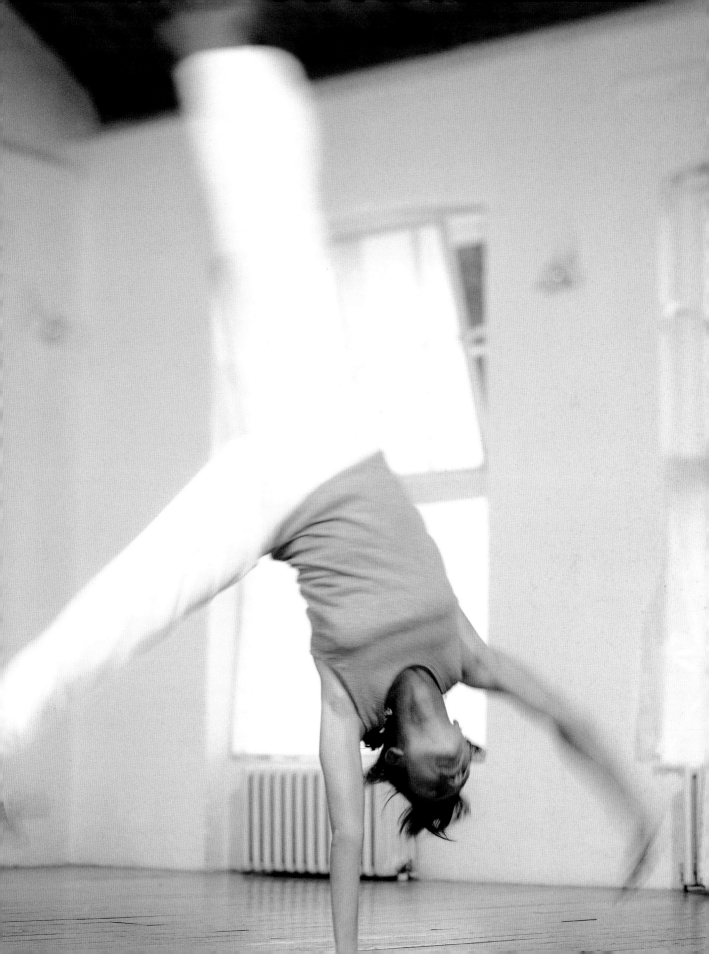

What you do in these 21 days

if you're 20-35...

Your fitness levels are potentially at an all-time high and you can still burn fat off quickly. So if you haven't been exercising, it's time to get off the sofa and start reclaiming your body's vitality and contours while your skin's supple enough to spring back into shape.

● Manage your stress levels. Concentrate on deep abdominal breathing during exercise.
● Build up strength and stamina through any additional moderate to fast aerobic sessions you enjoy: cycling, jogging, swimming (fast), rowing, cross training, squash or fitness classes are all ideal.
● Boost your brainpower at work. Seek out body/mind conditioning classes such as pilates, yoga or t'ai chi to improve concentration and create a lithesome, shapely body.

...35-50

A demanding lifestyle often puts exercise on the 'must do, haven't time' list. Fact is, you can't afford to leave it much longer, for as your body starts to slow with age so does your metabolism. If you've been relatively inactive until now, it's likely that you've been losing muscle tone and your body-fat percentage has been increasing. Exercise and good nutrition can turn it around.

● Focus. You don't have to look middle-aged. Fashion doesn't stop at 35. A trim healthy figure is rejuvenating inside and out, so keep moving.
● Boost your regime with any moderate aerobic exercise you can do at a brisk pace: swimming, cycling, dancing, tennis and so on.
● Work on cellulite. Drink more water, especially while exercising, to boost lymphatic drainage and reduce toxins. Exercise is key – but bump up your regime with lots of body brushing (see page 122) and your Nutrition programme (see chapter 1).

...or 50 and over

It's not too late to start, or pick up where you left off. Research shows exercising four times a week can reduce your risk of a heart attack by 38 per cent. It's rejuvenating too.

● Increase your strength, stamina and suppleness – all are vital to maintain as we age.
● Stick to 20 minutes for your aerobics, keep the pace light to moderate and don't push yourself. Swimming (slow), cycling (slow), badminton, gardening, all have a pace you can increase depending on fitness levels.
● Seek out body/mind conditioning classes, such as pilates, yoga or t'ai chi, for exercise that both stretches and relaxes.

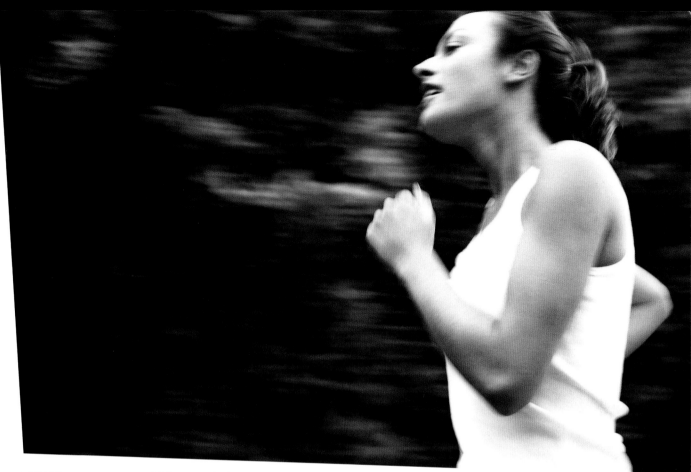

What you'll achieve

More energy Exercise increases your body's intake of oxygen, and that fuels your brain and every single cell in your body.

Look and feel younger Regular exercise is the ultimate anti-ageing weapon. It strengthens the heart and the lungs, lowers your resting heart-rate to combat stress, improves digestion, strength, stamina and suppleness, increases mental clarity, boosts circulation and stimulates the immune system. You really can live longer and feel younger.

Lighter mood Building regular exercise into your life is one of the best ways to lift your mood. Because exercise makes you breathe more deeply (and that's an antidepressant in itself), bringing more oxygen in to your body and energizing your very being, it makes you feel more alive. And exercise affects your pituitary gland too, which in turn releases the happy hormones known as endorphins.

Weight loss But you must follow the healthy eating plan in chapter 1 too. And this time you'll keep that weight off. Research consistently shows that it's only when you combine exercise and good nutrition that you get real weight-loss (and fitness).

Better body-image By exercising and eating healthily, you will automatically become more aware of your body. And you begin to learn to like what you see in the mirror. So, through positive thinking and a better fitness regime, dieting and bingeing should become less of an obsession.

Fun, yes fun Treating exercise more as a treat or indulgence than a burden will make the prospect more enjoyable.
● Choose a beautiful park or new destination to explore if you're walking.
● If you're 'not the exercising type', find some activity you can connect with to get motivated. Dancing, roller-blading, trampolining, for example, are all fun forms of aerobic exercise. Combine with a swim once a week, your brisk walks and early-morning stretch, and you're there. Think positive – you can fit a lot in and still have fun.

your fitness kit

Fitness/yoga mat

Comfort is important when you're doing floor exercises. You'll need a rolled-up towel too.

Stimulating essential oils

Black pepper*, cypress, eucalyptus, ginger and rosemary will all give you energy when you don't feel like working out. They also revitalize weary muscles post-workout. Dilute four to six drops of a stimulating oil in 10ml carrier oil (see page 220) before adding to the bath to ensure you don't 'overstimulate'.

*Avoid if you have high blood pressure.

Good sports bra

This is essential for comfort and support, especially while walking, when you need more support than you might appreciate.

Stretchy leotard top

Don't go for loose, baggy T-shirts to hide your figure – they just look like you're trying to hide your figure! Be proud, and stand tall. Wearing something more fitted during exercise makes it much easier to check your posture and improves your image.

Loose clothing

You need tracksuit bottoms and a fleece or light jacket for walking, and relaxed stretchy clothing for all yoga and pilates sequences.

Trainers

It's important to wear the right sports shoes for exercise. For walking, power-walking and running, buy trainers with high-density soles. To protect your knees and ankles, you need soles designed to absorb the intense impact of your feet as they pound the ground.

Yoga and pilates book or video

The brief stretches given in this book are typical, safe moves that everyone can do. However, if you have never done yoga or pilates before, I would suggest you buy a reputable book and/or video to give you the complete picture.

Water bottle

Buy a really nice one – it might inspire you to drink more.

For pilates

You will need a plump cushion (or soft ball) and a pair of 450g (1lb) dumbbells (or bottles of mineral water).

transformers

Feeling fit goes beyond feeling firm. It's about being healthy – a strong heart, efficient lungs and a clear head – and all these and more are within your reach with this 21-day exercise plan.

Morning stretch
(see pages 58–61)

Think of this as your kick-start to the day ahead. A yoga body stretch is the perfect way to begin each morning – one part meditation, one part stretching – and if there's one way to prepare you for busy meetings and a harassed day, this is it. Set your alarm 20 minutes earlier to avoid feeling rushed and pressurized before the day's begun.

Use to stretch and elongate muscle groups, strengthen the body, relieve stiffness, improve breathing, and calm and manage stress.

Midday aerobics
(see pages 62–7)

This can be any aerobic exercise that you enjoy – preferably a choice of three or four (see pages 66–7 for some favourites). I've focused on walking (at a normal-to-brisk pace) because it's simple and versatile. Easy to schedule into your midday, this might be a fast-paced walk to the sandwich bar – that one you love but usually can't be bothered to walk to. Or maybe you're on the hunt for new boots. Plan your route between several shops and keep moving. And it doesn't have to be at lunchtime (combine brisk walking with a mid-afternoon meeting and forget the bus or taxi). Think positively and think ahead. Use your daily planner and arrange your busy schedule, from meetings to the school run, to achieve a fitter, healthier you.

Use to fat burn, improve the cardiovascular system (get your heart pumping) and build stamina.

Evening tone-up
(see pages 68–73)

These five fantastic pilates moves use resistance to isolate and workout individual muscles. You could do them in the gym, but get yourself a comfortable mat and your bedroom/living-room floor is just as good. Twenty minutes will do, but if you can build up to 40 minutes by the end of the 21 days, all the better for you. Take each day as it comes. Do as much as you can in a session and then begin with the next exercise in the sequence next time you tone up. These exercises focus on those bits of the body we love the least – tummy, bottom, thighs, chest and backs of arms. Do them before eating supper so you can relax afterwards.

Use to tone specific areas that need attention and to lengthen and strengthen particular muscle groups.

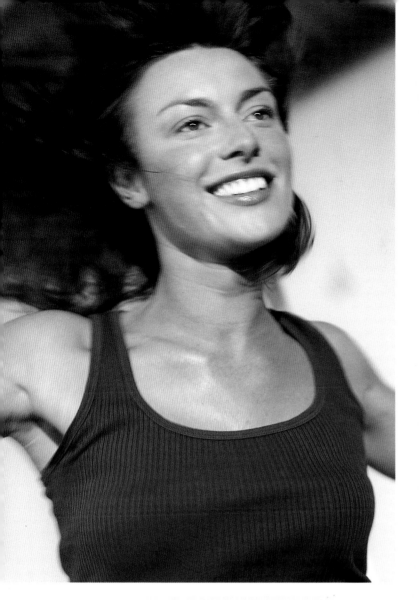

If you don't exercise regularly

Day 1-7 Your initial aim is to do a 20-minute yoga stretch each morning and then alternate your energy walk every other lunchtime with an evening pilates session. This means in your first week you should ideally manage to do 7 x 20min. early-morning stretches, 4 x 20min. lunchtime energy walks, and 3 x 20min. evening pilates sessions.

Boost it This is your intensive detox week on the Nutrition plan so you are beginning the Fitness plan gently .If you don't have much energy, try some of the tips offered to up energy levels and relieve headaches in chapter 1.

Day 8-14 In this week aim to increase the number of your midday walks (or aerobic sessions) to seven, keeping to your three 20-minute evening exercises.

Boost it By the middle of the week you should be feeling more energized, and your new regime (plus your new eating programme) will inspire you to improve on your fitness. If you feel inclined to cycle, play tennis with a friend, go dancing, skating or bowling, it all counts as aerobic exercise. So add it on top as a bonus, or swap with a walk one day.

Day 15-21 In your final week aim to increase the intensity of each type of exercise. Stretch just a little bit more with your yoga moves; go hill walking or over rough terrain. If you can, add in two more evening pilates sessions to focus and tighten specific muscles.

Boost it You should find that your energy levels are higher than you could possibly have imagined. If you're under 50 and feel comfortable extending the length of your midday and evening exercises to 30 or 40 minutes, the more the better.

If you exercise regularly

Simply increase the intensity of each exercise (i.e. hill climbs while walking, resistance on a bike, and longer sessions of up to 40 minutes rather than 20) if you can spare the time. This way you're working at your own fitness level, but can still see very real changes and benefits to your body and spirit.

Don't miss Gentle exercise is good for you. But always consult your doctor if you have a medical condition or are unused to exercise.

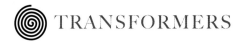
early morning stretch

The gentle stretches in these yoga poses will improve your posture and keep you strong but supple. Regular stretching plays a part in fitness because it helps to maintain the vital links between nerves and muscles. And that not only keeps our joints flexible but instills a state of calm.

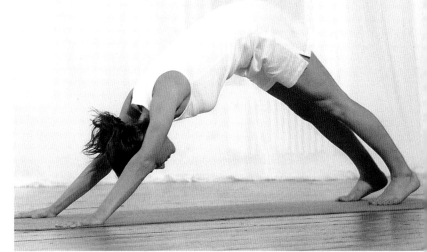

Yoga principles

Yoga is an ancient practice that combines relaxation and exercise for mind, body and spirit. It is considered an ideal way to reduce stress levels and restore the natural equilibrium of your body.

The postures (or asanas) are each gentle stretches which improve balance, strength and flexibility, coupled with correct breathing techniques. The movements are slow and controlled throughout the whole action of entering, holding and releasing each pose. They work on the entire body, including the internal organs, which are massaged by specific movements. Ideally you should first practise yoga in a beginner's class with a fully qualified instructor before trying anything from any book, although these simple poses are chosen with the complete beginner in mind. Approach them carefully and don't force the pace.

● Wear comfortable, loose clothing that doesn't restrict your movements.
● Go barefoot to avoid slipping.
● A soft mat is more comfortable on hard floors.

Breathing for yoga Breathing as you stretch helps to oxygenate your body, from your big toe to your brain, and that's how each yoga stretch releases tension.
● Breathe deeply using your abdominal muscles.
● Keep your breathing calm and even throughout.
● Take each exercise slowly and rhythmically.
● Never over-stretch your body until it hurts.

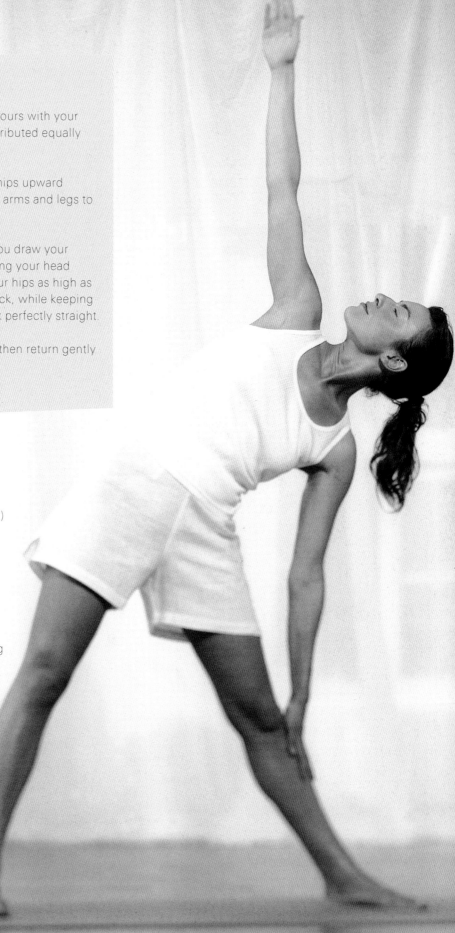

The down dog

1 Begin on the floor, kneeling on all fours with your toes curled under and your weight distributed equally between your hands and knees.

2 Inhale and as you exhale, lift your hips upward towards the ceiling, straightening your arms and legs to form an inverted V.

3 Press your heels into the floor as you draw your shoulder blades back and down, keeping your head between your shoulders. Aim to lift your hips as high as you can to take the tension off your back, while keeping your feet flat to the floor and your back perfectly straight.

4 Breathe freely for five breaths and then return gently to the kneeling position on all fours.

5 Repeat the whole movement twice.

The triangle

1 Stand with your feet almost 1m (3ft) apart and turn your left toes out to the side, keeping your right toes facing forward. Breathe in, and then out as you raise your arms to the sides until they are level with your shoulders.

2 Breathe in, and then out as you bend from your waist to the left, sliding your left hand down your left leg and extending your right arm upwards. Keep your legs straight and your torso facing forward.

3 Look up at your right hand as you take three deep breaths.

4 Relax into the standing pose. Reverse the position of your feet and repeat on the other side.

5 Repeat the whole movement.

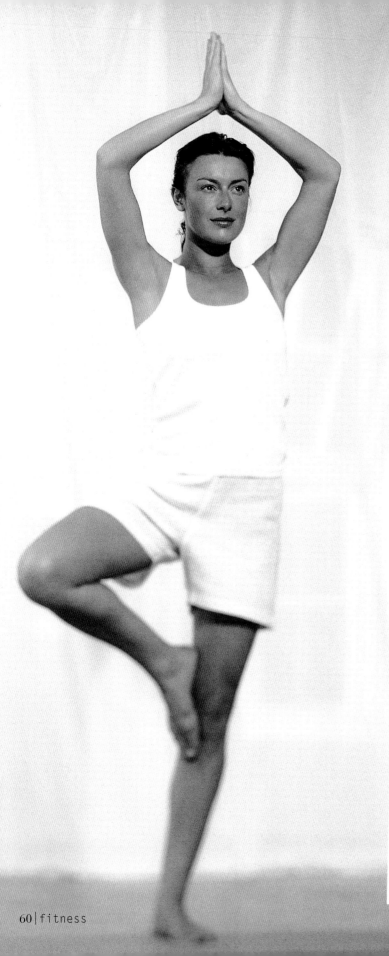

The butterfly

1 Sit on the floor with your back straight, your legs stretched in front of you and your shoulders relaxed. Breathe evenly and deeply through the remaining steps.

2 Bring the soles of your feet together in front of you and, using both your hands, draw your feet slowly and gently in toward your inner thighs.

3 Keeping your back straight and head up, try to feel a gentle stretch between your thighs as you lightly press your legs down toward the floor with your elbows. Hold the stretch for up to 30 seconds.

4 Relax and then repeat the whole movement twice.

The tree

1 Stand straight, feet together, arms by your sides, and breathe evenly.

2 Breathe in, and then out as you place all your weight on your left leg and raise your right leg, bending the knee and sliding the sole of the foot upward against the inner side of your left leg until it rests beside the left knee.

3 Place your palms together in a prayer position and then slowly raise your arms upward until they are over your head. Keep your elbows slightly bent. It helps your balance (which is tricky at first) if you focus on something straight ahead of you. Breathe calmly and rhythmically and try to stay in this position for up to 30 seconds.

4 Relax and repeat on your right leg.

5 Repeat the whole movement twice.

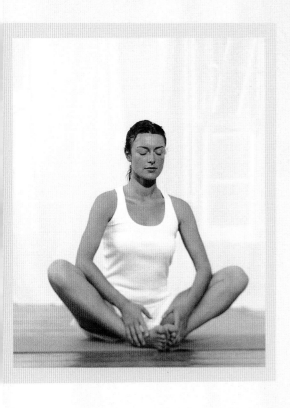

The spinal twist

1 Sit on the floor with both your legs stretched out in front of you.

2 Bending your left leg, move it over your right leg and place your left foot flat on the floor by the outer side of your right knee.

3 Place your left hand flat on the floor behind you, and then gently twist your upper body to the left to place your right hand flat on the floor on the outer side of your left leg. Your head should be in line with your left shoulder, keeping your shoulders straight.

4 Gently push your right elbow into your left knee and feel the stretch. Hold for six breaths.

5 Relax gently to the starting position and repeat on the other side.

6 Repeat this whole movement once again.

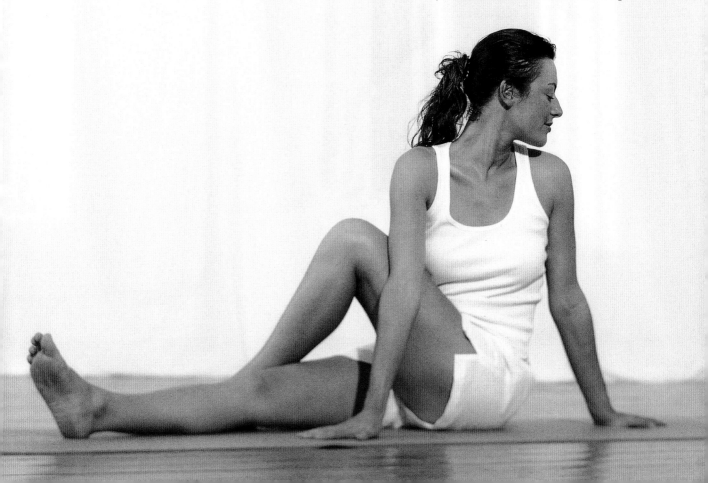

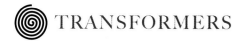

aerobic walking

The best exercise to lift your spirits and boost your detox is brisk walking. It can benefit every single one of us and it doesn't take a great deal of new-found skill because you've been doing it for years. It's great for weight loss too. And, don't forget, when you walk you're achieving something else - getting from a to b - so try making your exercise time work for you.

All the latest research reinforces the idea that moving at a regular, moderate pace – one at which you're working your muscles but are still able to hold a proper conversation although slightly breathless – maximizes your body's aerobic potential to burn fat. Exercises such as swimming and cycling are effective too, provided you don't go overdo it. Remember: it's important to work aerobic exercises at your own pace. Slow things down if you're working too hard.

Walking – or any other gentle aerobic exercise – also helps to eliminate toxins through the breath and through your skin, while encouraging your digestive system to work efficiently. So that's another boost for your Nutrition programme.

Remember
Week 1: 20 minutes x four times a week
Week 2: 20 minutes x seven times a week
Week 3: 20 minutes x seven times a week

How to check your heart rate
When trying to burn fat, keep your heart rate at about 60 per cent of your maximum heart rate – that usually means at around 115–130 beats per minute. It's easier to do this accurately with a pulse monitor, but if you're slightly breathless, not puffing, but warm with a bit of a sweat you're in the right zone. To calculate your heart rate while exercising, place your middle fingers on your wrist pulse and count the number of beats in 10 seconds. Multiple that figure by 6 and you have your heart rate per minute. Keep a check throughout, especially if you are new to exercise. Once your heart rate reaches the optimum zone, you need to maintain that pace for safe maximum effectiveness. Work any faster, and you're burning less fat.

Don't miss You can boost your metabolism with intermittent exercise just as you can from one uninterrupted, 20-minute walk.

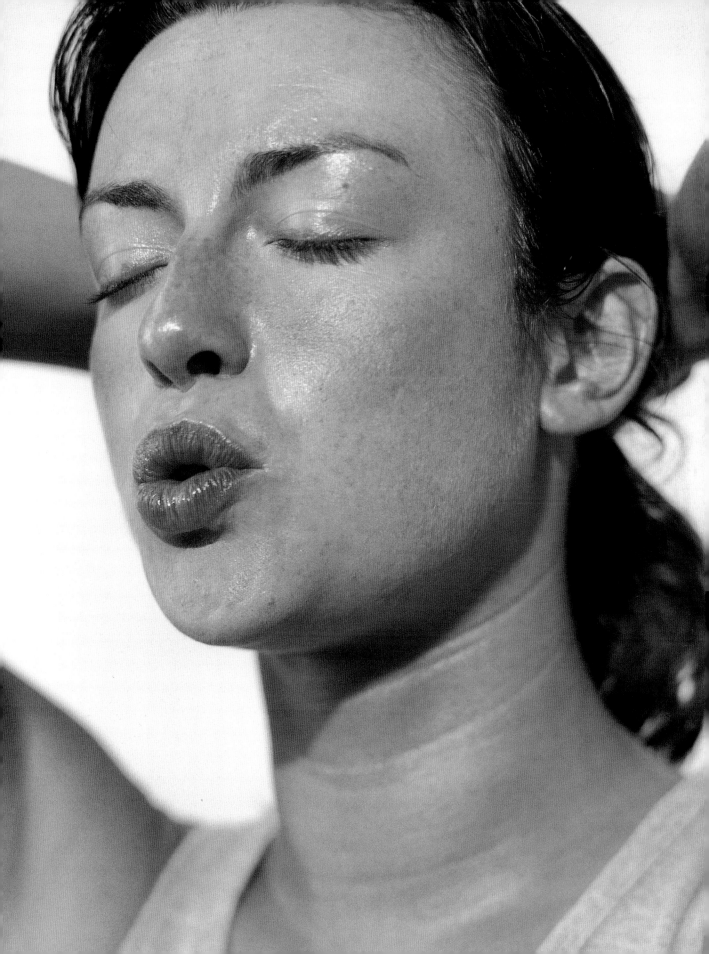

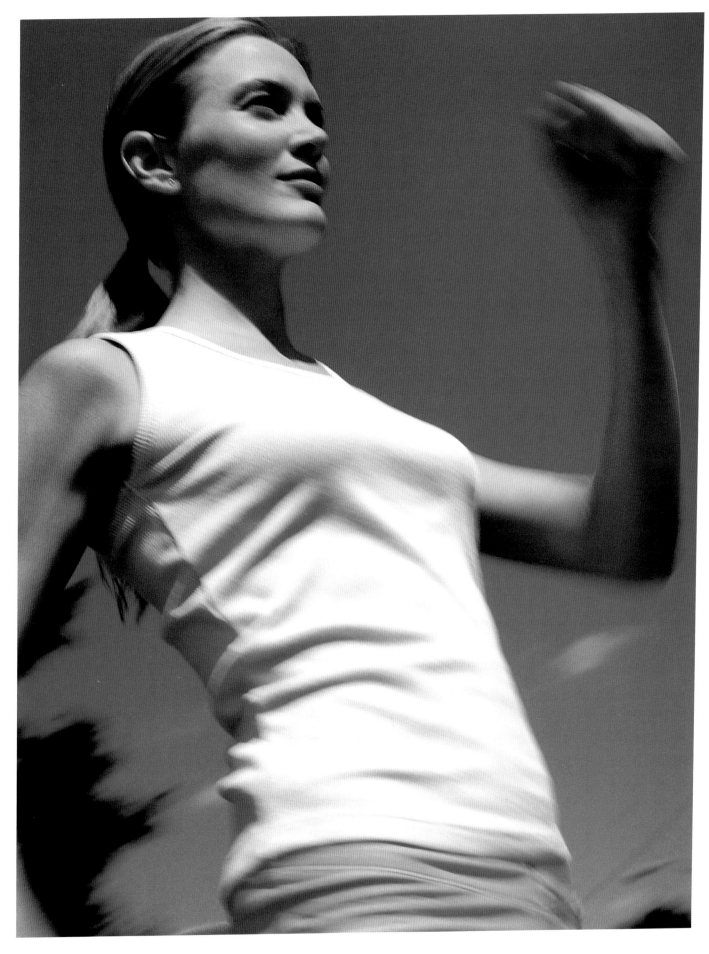

how to walk the walk

Warm up to your exercise – with a little walking – and stretch your leg muscles before and after. Stand with one leg behind the other, place your hands on your front knee, bend it, keep your back straight and feel the stretch in your straight, rear leg. Now reverse your position and give the other leg a stretch.

Your action

● Start by walking at an easy pace – slightly faster than you'd usually walk – for 6 minutes, to get your muscles and heart rate going.
● Then walk fast – as fast as you can (heel to toe, heel to toe) without ever losing your breath for 2 minutes.
● Now slow down to your easy walk for 2 minutes.
● Repeat the two 2-minute sequences twice more so that you do them three times in all.
● The final easy 2 minutes counts as your cool-down period.

Enjoy Choose an interesting route – in daylight and not isolated. Take a friend with you if you can. Not only will it ensure that you keep to your optimum pace, by talking, it's also safer and less boring. Encouragement too on bad-weather days. And don't forget your water bottle...

Your posture

1   With back straight and head held high, lift from your chest, and relax your shoulders (so the shoulder blades are retracted). This opens out the chest for better breathing.

2   Keep your chin level. It helps to imagine someone is pulling an imaginary string through the top of your head. Tug it every time you stoop.

3   Breathe. Keep it deep and controlled, in through your nose and out through your mouth.

4   Bend those elbows at 90 degrees (imagine you're holding ski poles) and swing your arms at a brisk pace. Give it some purpose.

5   You should walk heel to toe, rolling through to push off with the ball of your rear leg as you bring your other leg forward. Practise a little at first to make sure you're moving correctly.

6   Take shorter, quicker steps to work those buttocks and, if you can keep them squeezed as you walk, you'll strengthen your lower back too.

7   Keep your tummy held in as you walk (see pull navel to spine, page 68). This will dramatically transform the effect on your body, especially if you are using your arms too.

other aerobic exercise

You can swap any walk with some other moderate aerobic activity at any time. Just keep within your optimum aerobic heart rate. And always stretch your limbs before you exercise, especially for activities that involve sudden moves which may jolt your muscles and joints. Don't forget the water.

Swimming builds strength and stamina and is one of the best all-round exercises for everyone because, like walking, you can vary the pace to suit your fitness level and still achieve an excellent aerobic workout. Plus, because your body is suspended in water, you don't risk jolting your joints, making it suitable for every age.

● Backstroke tightens the abdominal muscles, tones the legs and upper arms, and burns off the most calories (up to 275 calories in 20 minutes) because it is such a complete body workout.
● Freestyle boosts body alignment and improves the whole cardiovascular system.
● Breaststroke strengthens your upper arms and tones the chest and inner thighs.

Cycling improves your co-ordination, stamina and muscle strength, and tones legs, hips and buttock muscles brilliantly. Always start slowly and gradually increase until you feel warm and slightly out of breath. Keep at this pace even when changing the gradient, but don't over-exercise or you'll burn less fat.

● Ensure your seat and handle bars are in the correct position for you. Your legs should be almost straight when the pedals are at their lowest position. Don't slouch – keep yourself upright.
● If you're cycling on the roads, wear a protective helmet and know your Highway Code. Avoid cycling in areas that are congested with traffic (or wear a mask) or too many pedestrians. Wide-open spaces are best – then you don't have to stop.

Don't underestimate any activity – just moving burns a few calories. Now you need to channel those moves into effective 20-minute slots so you burn off more.

Rowing is fantastic exercise once you get into the habit, especially for those who have a competitive streak since you can race against the equipment or against others.

● Keep your back straight, head up, shoulders relaxed, arms and legs straight out.
● Breathe in before you move, and breathe out as you pull the ropes. Get into a regular rhythm and pace, and breathe calmly and continuously. If you get short of breath, slow the pace.
● Tuck your tummy right in as you move for the maximum effect – it supports your back too.

Tennis & Squash boost your entire cardiovascular system, strengthen arms and legs, and shape the waist. Tennis is less intense than squash, though it depends with whom you play.

● You'll develop your own individual style in either sport, but I suggest a short series of professional lessons to give you the right moves.
● Remember that pre-game stretch to help prevent hamstring injuries resulting from sudden moves, and give support to your knees if you have a weakness.
● Always wear good trainers and light clothing.

Skipping is a great way to tone up and very convenient, if, of course, you have a skipping rope – adult size. It tones thighs, calves and buttocks, gives your body one of the most effective cardiovascular workouts and improves your co-ordination.

● Stand upright, head held high and tummy pulled in.
● Aim to breathe calmly and evenly throughout.
● Start off with just 5 minutes – it's harder than you might think. Build up to 20 with practice.

Any form of dance, from

ballet and ballroom to belly, improves all-round fitness. You use all sorts of different muscle groups, depending on which type of dance. But most of all it improves muscle tone, flexibility, co-ordination and posture. And the faster the pace, the more calories you'll burn.

Gardening counts

Preferably the digging kind rather than the pruning kind!

WHAT YOU BURN OFF

Aerobic activity	Maximum calories in 20 minutes
FIT	
Skipping	260 CALORIES
Squash	260 CALORIES
Cycling (brisk)	240 CALORIES
Swimming (moderately fast)	230 CALORIES
Kick boxing	210 CALORIES
Rowing	200 CALORIES
Skating (in line)	160 CALORIES
Tennis	160 CALORIES
Low-impact aerobics class	130 CALORIES
& FUN	
Dancing	110 CALORIES
Gardening	110 CALORIES
Swimming (slow)	90 CALORIES
Playing with kids in the park	80 CALORIES
Bowling	70 CALORIES
Shopping with heavy bags	60 CALORIES
Kissing	45 CALORIES
Housework	35 CALORIES

Figures based on a 63.5kg (10st) woman

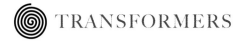
early evening tone-up

Pilates stretches (and so elongates) the muscles, rather than building them up, working against resistance and without gravity, so that each exercise is safe for all ages and levels of fitness without any risk of strain or injury.

The pillow Inner thighs

1 Lie on your back, your head resting on a rolled-up towel, and place a cushion (or soft ball) between your knees. Your knees should be bent, feet flat on the floor, hip-width apart.

2 Check your tailbone (or sitting bone) is on the floor and your feet are parallel. If they tend to roll outward, you may need to place a tennis ball between your ankles too so you'll have to concentrate on keeping that in place as well.

3 Breathe in and pull navel to spine. Breathe out as you squeeze the cushion firmly between your knees (as shown) and tighten your pelvic-floor muscles.

4 Continue to squeeze the cushion, using your inner thigh muscles NOT your hips for a count of 10. Lengthen through your spine as you squeeze.

5 Repeat the whole movement nine times.

Pilates principles

This body-conditioning technique was created over forty years ago by Joseph Pilates, a German athlete. With elements of t'ai chi, yoga and the Alexander technique, pilates works by combining strict posture and breathing techniques to produce greater body awareness, self-discipline and inner relaxation. Each movement is smooth and rhythmical. You should never strain or feel pain.
● Wear loose, comfortable clothing.
● Keep feet bare or in socks.
● You need some simple equipment for this session: a plump cushion (or soft ball), a tennis ball (optional) and a couple of 450g (1lb) dumbbells (or bottles of mineral water).

Breathing for pilates Correct breathing works your lungs and heart, boosts blood circulation and makes it much easier to control tension.
● Breathe in before each movement
● Breathe out during the movement.

Pull navel to spine You'll find this instruction throughout the section. It's used in pilates exercise to ensure that you maximize each movement. It simply means pull your tummy in from your belly button as far as you can – imagining it can touch your spine helps. You should hold your tummy in like this throughout the whole movement while breathing as described above.

Because you hold your tummy in the entire time, pilates is the best exercise for a flatter tummy. Forget all those old fast-paced, sit-up tummy exercises. If you sit from lying down, you may strain yourself. Research now shows that the smaller, slower and more targeted the movement, the better the exercise.

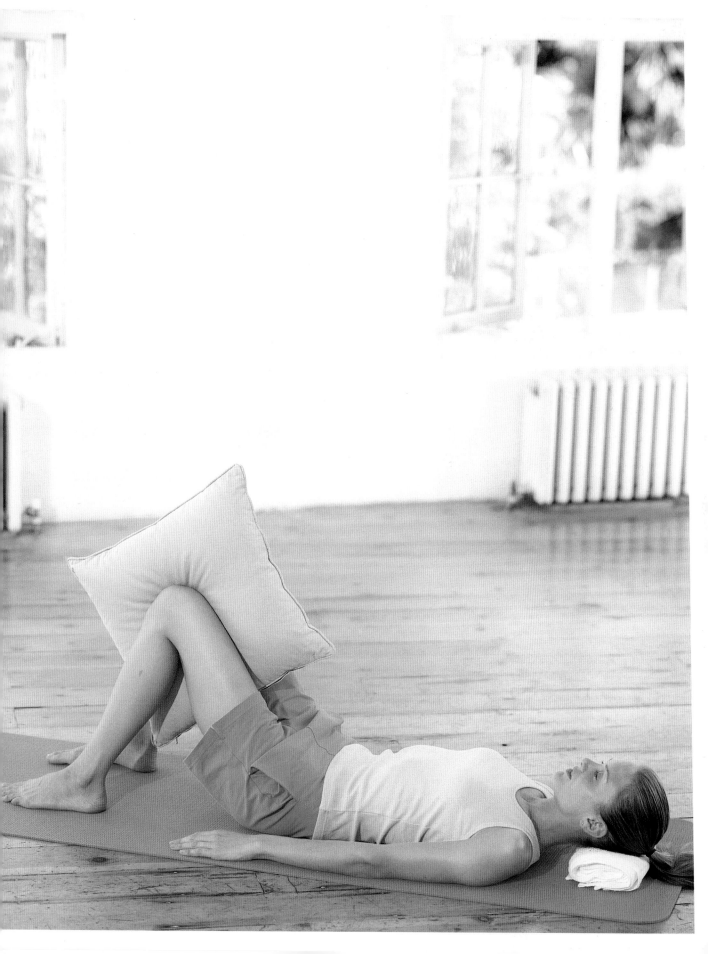

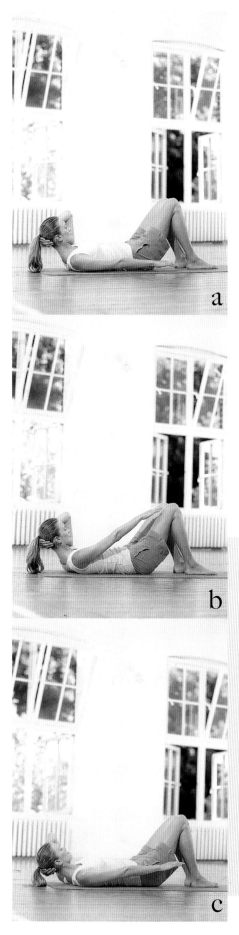

a

b

c

The single-leg stretch Abdominals

1   With your head on a folded towel so your chin is parallel to the floor, lie on your back, your knees bent and your feet hip-width apart. Keep your toes parallel, back flat and tailbone tucked under.

2   Breathe in and pull navel to spine. Breathe out as you bring both knees up toward your chest and place your hands on your outer calves. Keep your toes relaxed and pointing downward (as shown, a).

3   Breathe in and then breathe out as you curl your head and upper body off the floor (as shown, b). They remain raised off the floor throughout all the following steps.

4   Breathe in and then out as you stretch your left leg out until it is straight, making a 45-degree angle with the floor, while your right knee remains closer to your chest with both hands lightly holding the knee (as shown, c).

5   Breathe in as you straighten your right leg to make that 45-degree angle with the floor, and then out as you bring your left knee in toward your chest, lightly holding the knee (as shown, d).

6   Repeat the whole movement ten times. The action should glide from one leg to the other, and you breathe out as one leg is stretched away and in as the other leg is pulled in.

Oblique curls Waist

1   Lie on your back on the floor with your knees bent and feet flat. Place your left hand under your head for support. Your right arm is at your side, palm down

2   Breathe in and pull navel to spine. Breathe out as you slowly raise your left side, moving it up and towards the right (as shown, a). It helps to increase the lift if you imagine someone is pushing up from under your shoulder blade. Let your tummy muscles do the work rather than your left arm. (If you feel tension in your neck, you can give it more support by using both hands behind your head.)

3   Breathe in as you raise your right arm and out as you stretch to touch your left knee (as shown, b). Slowly lower your arm to the floor (as shown, c).

4   Do the whole movement ten times on each side.

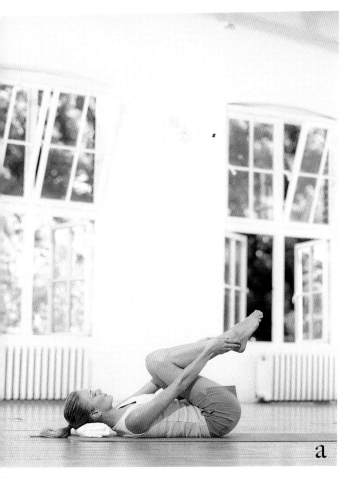

a

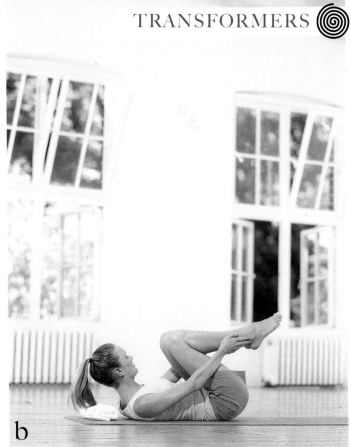

b

c

d

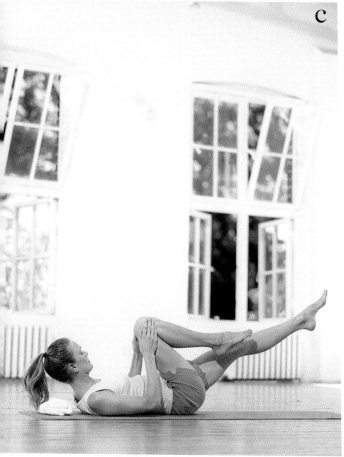

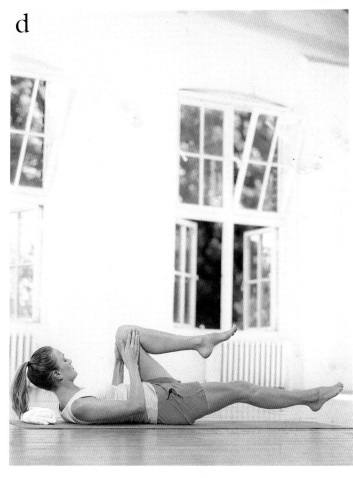

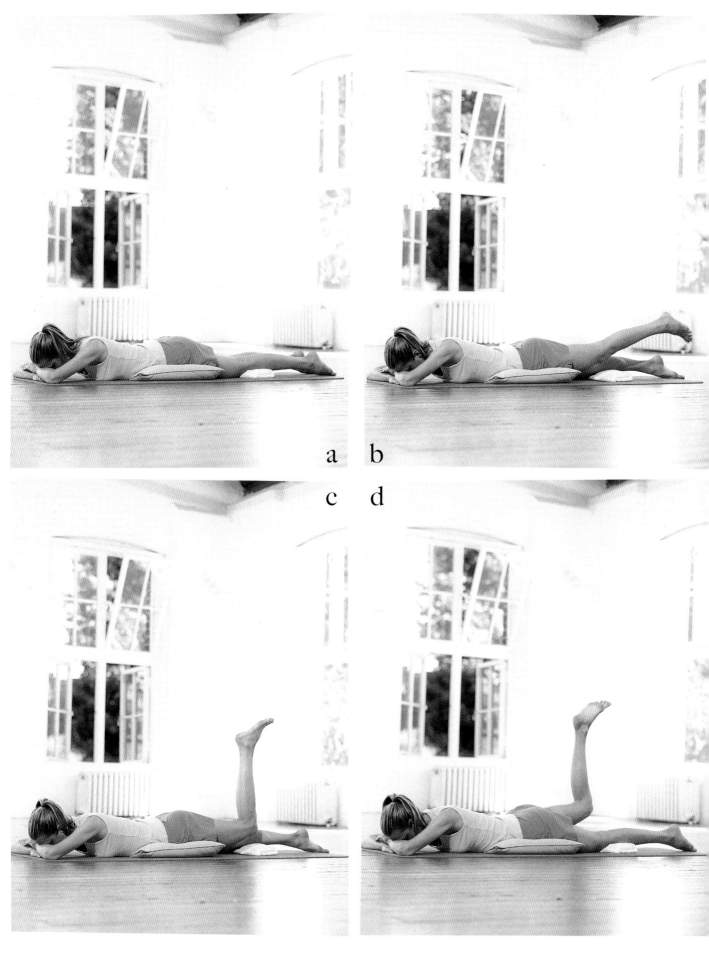

a b

c d

Twos Arms & shoulders

In a pilates studio you'd do the exercise lying on a
narrow bench with your arms dangling over the
side, but this version can be done at home.

1   Stand with your feet hip-width apart, your
shoulders relaxed and your back flat.

2   Holding a weight in each hand (either 450g/1lb
dumbbells or bottles of water), bend your elbows
and bring your arms up to chest height, hands
facing one another in the middle (as shown, a).

3   Breathe in and pull navel to spine. Breathe out
as you slowly semi-circle your arms out to the
sides, keeping them slightly bent at the elbows and
level with your chest to a count of 10. As you move
your arms out to the sides, concentrate on working
the muscles in your upper arms to resist the
movement (as shown, b). This way you focus on
the muscle you are working.

4   Breathe in and breathe out as you bring your
arms back in front of you.

5   Do the whole movement ten times, keeping the
action flowing without pause.

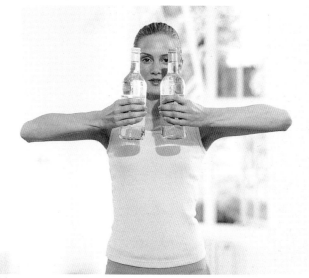

a

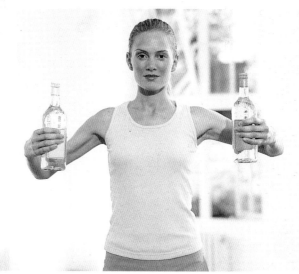

b

The diamond press Buttocks

1   With a pillow under your tummy to support the curve or lumbar region of
the spine and a small, rolled towel under your knees, lie face down on the floor
with your head resting on your forearms (as shown: a). Imagine your tailbone
being pulled towards your feet but keep them relaxed.

2   Breathe in and pull navel to spine. Breathe out as you squeeze your buttocks
together and slowly raise your lower left leg until it's upright (as shown, b & c),
relaxing your foot to use the calf muscles. Hold for a count of 4 and release.

3   Repeat, raising and lowering your left leg nine times.

4   Using your right leg (as shown: d), repeat the whole movement.

Move a little more than you did yesterday Hide the remote control. Take every opportunity for a brisk walk: post a letter, get some air, buy the morning papers and use those stairs.

Dance Turn the music up and wiggle away to three or four songs.

Work with your body rhythms
Research shows that morning exercisers stick to it more than those who exercise at the end of a day. So fit in any additional exercise early when your energy is high. And, if you need a boost before your early evening session, inhale a little peppermint oil to help you focus (see page 220).

Extra-easy aerobics Take the bus to work and get off one or two stops earlier (make sure you've built in the time to do this). Your 20-minute power walk could be done by 9.30am.

Avoid dehydration while exercising Drink one or two glasses of water an hour before exercise. Then sip every 15 minutes or so as you work out.

Eating and exercise? An orange or kiwi (both high in vitamin C) before your workout gives you a boost of energy. But if you've eaten a big meal, the only exercise to do is walking.

Missed a routine? That housework counts as a workout in itself (see the chart on page 67). Put a little extra effort in and you're there.

Preventing stiffness? Give yourself a great body scrub while you shower after exercising. Pay attention to the muscles you've just worked too.

Ouch If you've used muscles that haven't been worked for some time, they may well feel stiff and sore. Add one drop each of black pepper*, ginger, eucalyptus and cypress pure essential oil to 10ml (1 tbsp) jojoba, almond or grapeseed carrier oil (see page 220) and massage.
* Avoid if you have high blood pressure.

Improve your posture Stretch and stand tall. You've just taken 2.25–4.5kg (5–10lbs) off your body. Poor posture not only reflects 'a sad old me' image, it can also affect digestion and the functioning of all your internal organs.

Stand up straight Pull your tummy in. (Weak tummy muscles are responsible for most back problems.) Keeping your head level, let your chin find its natural position. It helps to imagine your head as a ball, held aloft on a fountain (your spine). Straighten your shoulders by scrunching them up to your ears and then letting them relax down again. Standing straight adds to your height too.

If you have a tense neck Slowly turn your head to the left as far as you can stretch and hold for a count of 10. Then slowly turn back to face the centre, drop your head down to your chest, hold for 10 and bring it back up again. Now turn your head to the right as far as you can stretch and hold for 10. Repeat five times.

keeping it going

Focus on the positive

You've achieved so much. Well done. And the good news is that you'll find it much easier to maintain your fitness programme than it was when you began three weeks ago. So don't come to a halt now that the magical 21 days is over.

● Learn to make fitness second nature to you, even if it's only because you know it does you good.

● Try something new. This is your chance to arrange a salsa class, go skating, belly dancing or hiking. A change in any established body routine can make a difference to your vitality.

● Find a fitness buddy to join you for classes or on bike rides. Not letting the other one down is always a great motivator.

● Gradually increase the intensity of your walks rather than the length. Choose a hill walk if possible, carry a half-full back pack, or up the pace, provided that your breathing remains even and your heart rate isn't beyond your fat-burning zone.

● Buy a heart-rate monitor to help you workout at the right pace.

Seek balance

Relax to recharge Join a local yoga class or buy a good video – it's one of the best workouts for total flexibility. While aerobic exercise has proven training effects, yoga, t'ai chi and other mind/body exercises also offer energizing effects and are anti-stress.

Vary your workout Cross training – swapping cycling, say, with swimming and then rowing and walking – not only varies the pace and uses different muscle groups to keep you really toned all over, it also makes exercise much more appealing. Swap around: anything you enjoy that's aerobic and works within your heart-rate capacity is doing you good.

Choose a better path

● What's your motivation? If you have a fitness goal, you'll not only improve your physique, it'll get you more motivated in other areas of your life too.

● Fit as much moderate exercise into your schedule as you feel you can. Don't get stressed about it, but the virtue of moderate-pace exercise is that anyone can achieve it.

● Avoid the energy zappers: stress, depression, anxiety, anaemia, poor diet, sedentary lifestyle, dehydration, overwork, eating on the run, lack of fresh air, insufficient sleep, emotional strain and negative thoughts.

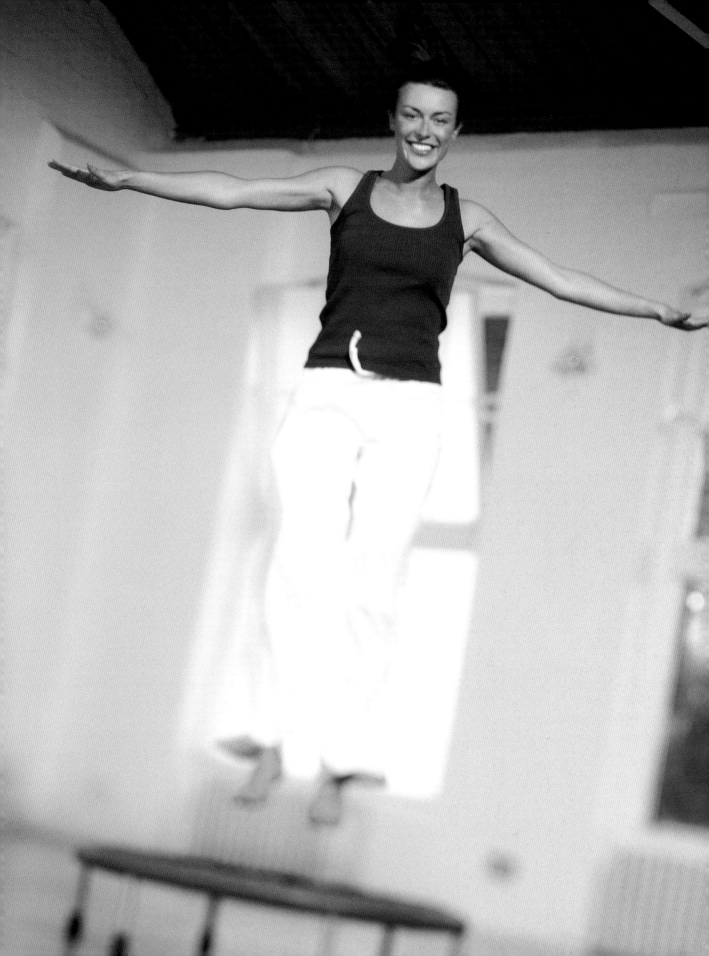

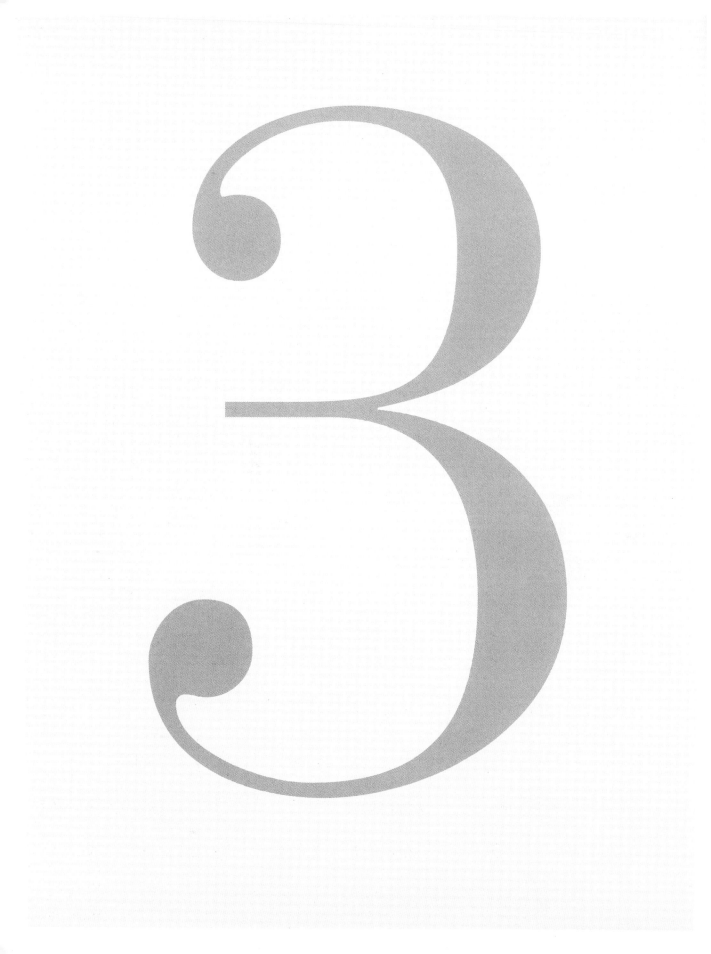

21 DAYS TO RADIANT SKIN

Radiance comes from within. Your skin is just the surface with which you face the world. But care for it, love it, and you care for your inner being.

Your skincare programme

The aim couldn't be simpler: you're going to improve your skin and delay the effects of ageing. Because if there's one thing that will make you look and feel like a new you it's softer, smoother skin. When your skin looks good, you radiate health and vitality. And before you say wrinkles are wrinkles and you can't turn back the clock, it's worth considering that perceptions of skin quality owe more to texture and tone than line and wrinkle.

THE POSITIVE NEWS IS THAT SKIN RENEWS ITSELF – YOU JUST NEED TO PUSH IT ALONG A LITTLE.

Why does skin age?
Young skin is plump, vibrant and renews itself every 21 days without help. But beyond even age 25, you need to fool it into acting young again. Everything slows down. Less oil is produced so skin feels drier. Cell renewal takes longer so skin becomes dull, uneven and starts to let crucial amounts of moisture sneak out. And then, in time, under the consistent assault of ultraviolet (UV) rays and the elements, your springy skin becomes slack, thin and crepey.

But ageing is a choice we make
If you protect your skin every day and boost its natural renewal process, you can encourage dead skin cells to fall off more quickly, making way for fresh new cells, and that's what keeps your skin looking vibrant. Only 20 per cent of lines are certain: the rest is down to the way you live your life.

Enemies within and without
Sitting in front of VDUs for hours on end, copious cups of coffee and sugary snacks, eating on the run, coupled with the stress and pace of life – all attack our skin from the inside. Then there are the external threats. Indoors, it's central heating and air conditioning, which quickly dehydrate skin leaving it super-sensitive. Go outside and, whatever the weather, exposure to UVA rays 365 days of the year further dehydrates skin and causes free-radical damage deep down, which in turn leads to premature ageing. And, there's atmospheric pollution – smoke and traffic fumes... You're exposed to it ALL.

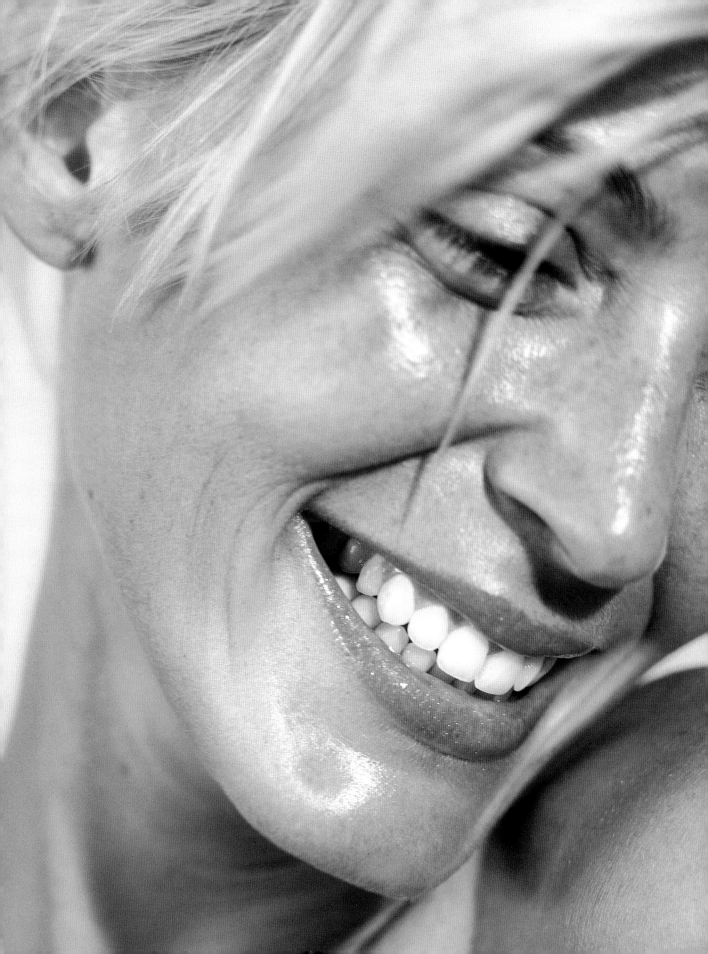

What you do in these 21 days

if you're 20-35...

Act now to keep your skin at its best. If you've been a sun-worshipper, exposure to sunlight will already have reduced its elasticity, leading to premature fine lines and wrinkles. Many fine lines are also due to dryness and a poor lymphatic system.

● Protect your face from UV rays and pollution. Experts insist that damage prevention at this age is the best anti-ageing skincare tactic. Choose a broad-spectrum sunscreen that gives equal, even protection against UVA and UVB (see page 85).
● Remove your make-up before bed. Cleanse and moisturize twice a day. Use beautifying treatments once a week.
● Improve your diet, drink plenty of mineral water and find time for relaxation.
● Don't skimp on your vitamin intake, especially if you have a demanding lifestyle. Remember to top up with additional iron, vitamin-B complex, vitamins C and E (all found in a multi-vitamin and mineral supplement) and evening primrose oil: these make a real difference to your skin and wellbeing.

...35-50

Your skin may have lost up to 30 per cent of its elasticity, but you can make it feel softer and look more radiant. This is the time to reduce stress, which always shows on your skin first.

● Moisturize – look for creams containing antioxidants as free-radical damage speeds up now, resulting in drier skin and patchy, uneven pigmentation. Invest in a regular facial as a skin booster.
● Gently exfoliate once a week – essential because cell renewal is beginning to slow down.
● Delay the ageing process with clean living! Poor nutrition, sun exposure and life have damaged the collagen and elastin fibres that act like a springy mattress under the skin's surface, causing a significant loss of elasticity.

...50 and over

After the menopause, skin takes longer to renew itself. It holds less moisture and lines becomes more noticeable – not just around the eyes but around the mouth, the cheeks and the throat, too.

● Moisturize more than ever. Don't stick with one all-purpose moisturizer. Layer products designed to do different jobs.
● Be gentle. Research shows that over-zealous exfoliation of mature skin can thin the protective outer layer too much, making skin more sensitive.
● Remember: regular exercise and a sensible diet are still the most effective beauty regime.
● Keep your face out of the sun. Age spots (also called sun or pigmentation spots) are caused by accumulated sun damage.

What you'll achieve

Suppleness   Your skin will look and feel more stretchy and springy up to six hours after applying moisturizer in the morning.

Softness   There will be a smoother, softer feel to any areas of dryness or irritation.

Evenness   Areas of irregular pigmentation will appear less obvious, and there'll be a reduction in blackheads and whiteheads.

Assessing your skin

The cosmetics industry likes to label you and your skin – it makes things easier. But it doesn't feel easy when you're confronted by 12 different face creams from one company alone. And if you don't understand your own skin type, how can you determine which products to use? So learn how to assess your own skin, and remember: skin changes through the years – just as your environment, life and health change over time.

How does your skin look? Be objective. Look closely in daylight, examine each pore and fine line. Touch it – is it even and smooth? Pinch the cheeks and chin – does it still spring back quickly? Is it puffy first thing? Do you have dark circles or blocked pores indicating a toxic build-up within? (See face mapping on page 106 for further assessment.)

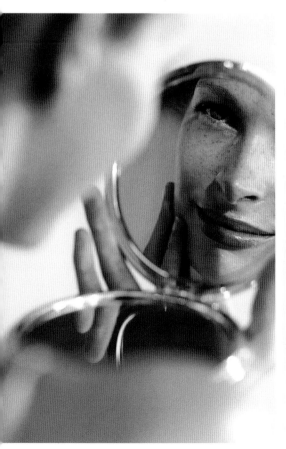

Sensitive skin is fine and translucent, and easily develops early fine lines and spider veins. It's quick to become irritated by perfume, active skincare ingredients, allergens such as lanolin, pollutants and poor care, resulting in redness and itchiness.
● Use gentle fragrance-, alcohol- and lanolin-free products where possible. Stick to plant oils and avoid products containing petrochemicals or other synthetic ingredients. Restrict face scrubs to once every two or three weeks. Always wear a broad-spectrum sunscreen (see page 85): high in levels of titanium dioxide or zinc oxide.

Dry skin is fine and has a close texture. It may feel tight, flaky and easily develop fine lines and early wrinkles, or may simply be more mature. It needs good protection against all weathers.
● Avoid soap and use gentle, creamy cleansers, alcohol-free toners, moisturizing cream and broad-spectrum sun protection. Always use a night cream and a moisturizing face mask.

Normal skin is near perfect. It's soft, finely textured and apparently poreless. It doesn't dry, flake, become oily or spotty. But it's hard to keep it that way.
● Use gentle products on a regular basis to maintain skin texture and protect from UV with a broad-spectrum sunscreen.

Combination skin is the most common type. The classic T-zone – forehead, nose and chin – is shiny, while the skin around the eyes, cheeks and neck is dry. There are more sebaceous glands in the T-zone than on other parts of the face and it's this concentration of over-active glands (see oily skin, below) that is the cause of that oily zone.
● Use products for oily skin only on the T. Cleanse all over and then concentrate moisturizer on the cheeks. Once a week, focus your face scrub on the T-zone, and use a gentle face mask for all-over cleansing. Don't forget the broad-spectrum sunscreen.

Oily skin looks shiny and is prone to spots and blemishes. It's due to high levels of testosterone which increase oil production (or sebum) in the skin. The skin has a thicker texture and may have enlarged and blocked pores with a tendency to blackheads.
● Gentle cleansing is paramount. Over-zealous cleansing stimulates the oil glands to produce even more oil, and leaves skin open to infection. And that can lead to 'problem skin'. Choose a mild pH-balanced soap or cleanser (wash–off is better), toner and oil-free moisturizer. Use a face scrub once a week, along with a deep-cleansing mask and a facial steam. Even oily skin needs broad-spectrum sun protection.

your skincare kit

Indispensable

ALL THE ITEMS REQUIRED FOR THE MUST-DO
DAILY TRANSFORMERS ARE LISTED. ONCE
YOU'VE DECIDED WHICH BEAUTIFIERS AND
BOOSTERS MOST APPEAL TO YOU, PREPARE A
PERSONAL CHECKLIST OF OTHER ESSENTIALS
YOU'LL NEED, SO YOU HAVE EVERYTHING TO
HAND WHEN YOU MOST NEED IT.

Cleanser

Choose between a creamy or rinse-off
formula, whichever you and your skin
prefer. Check pages 83 and 86 if you're not
sure. Use separate make-up removers for
eyes and for face to cleanse properly.

Essential oils

For dry, mature and sensitive skins, rose
and neroli are invaluable with a facial
massage (see page 100). Unnecessary for
oily or combination skin, use a skin serum.
Rose also combines with vitamin E oil (see
skin oils) for a conditioning lip mask.

Eye care

Everyone needs moisturizer around their
eyes. Some use a cream (fine eye lines
and/or dry skin) or a gel (oilier and/or young
skin), or even both. But keep checking – a
gel may not be rich enough for fine lines, or
a cream may be too heavy at night. Stay
aware of how your skin reacts to what you
put on it – and what you leave off.

Good mirror

You need to be able to view your skin well,
preferably in daylight so you can see
everything. If that's not possible, get a hand
mirror and look at your skin by the window.
Use it before and after doing your basic
daily am regime. Check for clean pores, dry
patches and fine lines.

Lip balm or petroleum jelly

Essential for keeping the fine, delicate skin
on your mouth smooth, soft and less prone
to chapping, apply a lip balm frequently
throughout the day.

Moisturizer

Every skin needs moisture. Even oily skin, which has plenty of oil, needs water from a basic moisturizer. Choose day and night creams based on your skin type and your age requirements. Turn to page 87 for a quick run-through.

Skin oils

A selection of skin oils, such as almond, avocado, borage, jojoba, vitamin E and wheatgerm oil, give extra nourishment to dry, dehydrated skins. Select your favourite – each one has a particular aroma – and use either alone for massage (face and body) or mix together in equal quantities and store in a coloured glass jar in a cool, dark place. Used with potent aromatherapy essentail oils for therapy and fragrance, they are known as 'carrier' oils (see page 220).

Skin serum

Use day or night, under moisturizer for day if your skin's dry, or as a lighter alternative to night cream (especially for normal to oily skins – your skin gets to breathe and will feel less clogged).

Sun protection

Rated as the single most effective anti-ageing product you can use, provided you do so on a daily basis, choose a broad-spectrum sunscreen with a minimum sun protection factor (SPF) of 15. Broad-spectrum products evenly protect from UVA (the ageing ray, around morning till night, all year round, and penetrates deep into the skin) and from UVB (the burning ray and strongest in sunny weather).

Makes a big difference

Facial exfoliator This makes the difference between good skin and great skin. Choose between a 'smooth-bead' scrub (rather than one made from irregular particles, such as walnuts, that can scratch) and an enzyme exfoliator that dissolves dead skin cells rather than rubbing them off.

Face mask Fantastic for all skin types, there's a mask for every occasion, day or night. Turn to page 97 to find out which are best for your skin and how to use them.

Muslin cloth Buy a 20cm (8in) strip of butter muslin, cut into four and stitch the edges so they wear well. They can be used daily to buff the skin.

Rosewater As a natural, skin-refreshing toner, rosewater is great – but not essential. However, if you use a creamy cleanser and need that 'clean feeling' afterwards, this is the mildest toner to use that won't over-stimulate your skin.

transformers

Proper cleansing, protecting and nourishing can dramatically enhance your skin's vitality. Advances in skincare are now so sophisticated that they are designed to give skin at any age all the help it needs: boosting cell renewal, increasing protection from the elements and fighting off free-radical damage with skin-energizing vitamins, herbs and plants. The quick route to better-looking skin is based on two essentials.

Cleansing

Daily cleansing brightens skin fast. Clear pores and a brighter complexion say youth and vitality – so don't skimp on it.

Soap is fine if it's pH-balanced and your skin feels comfortable after rinsing. Problems arise when it isn't removed well. Soap mixed with water can leave a residue that clings to skin, resulting in a dry, taut feeling.

Soap-free, rinse-off cleansers are pH-balanced, clean well and are removed easily. These suit all skin types.

Cleansing creams which are wiped away with a tissue or cotton wool are generally preferred by those with very dry or mature skin and are a gentle option for delicate skin.

Make-up removers contain special ingredients designed to remove the stubborn traces that your facial cleanser just won't shift. So, if you wear make-up daily, removers for face and eyes become essential for cleaner, brighter skin.

Take things easy Never be over-zealous when cleansing. A good product will leave your skin clean without rubbing. If your skin is acne-prone, go gentler still on cleansing and avoid exfoliants. Acne can be an inflammatory response, and cleansers and exfoliators that are too abrasive may irritate further. Look for a very mild cleanser with an anti-bacterial agent. If you have sensitive skin, it's worth seeking out sensitive-skin ranges that minimize potential skin irritants and include soothing botanical extracts

Fast track Do it in the shower. Speed up your morning skincare regime by washing your face with a rinse-off cleanser as you shower. Simple but it saves a vital 2–3 minutes first thing.

Moisturizing

Moisturizers range from a basic day cream to action-packed antioxidant, protective, preventative and anti-ageing creams. But their basic function remains the same: to act as a barrier and keep moisture in the skin.

Day creams come in several forms. Rich, textured creams suit normal, dry and mature skin. Light lotions are suitable for normal or sensitive skin. Oil-free creams or lotions suit combination or oily skin: you need moisture to plump the cells, but hold the oil.

Night creams are essential too. Skincare experts say skin cells renew themselves faster while you sleep so this is a good time to apply a treatment cream. If you use a night cream and find that your skin looks oily and congested by morning, you probably don't need it. Leave it off for a few days and see if your skin improves. If it does, swap to a lighter serum instead. These gel creams absorb more quickly and are less likely to clog your pores.

Eye products may sound like indulgence but the skin here is fragile and needs individual treatment. Eye creams and gels are lightweight and designed not to irritate your eyes.

Advanced anti-ageing treatment creams with ingredients such as retinol (vitamin A derivative), alpha-hydroxy acids (AHAs) and enzyme technology are recommended only if your skin isn't sensitive, you're over 35 or your skin is sun damaged. These are often designed to be used at night as the ingredients can be UV sensitive.

Keep checking Regularly assess your skin over the next three weeks to see how it improves with your higher intake of omega-3 oil. If you find that it regularly breaks out or is prone to blocked pores or blackheads, you probably have oily skin and should switch to an oil-free moisturizer. Likewise, if your skin is especially dry, you need to up your water intake and change your moisturizer to one that attracts more water to your skin with humectants (such as hyaluronic acid).

Sun protection Dermatologists recommend using a SPF of at least 15 (this provides you with up to 94 per cent UV protection for 15 times longer before your skin reddens). The higher the SPF, the better the protection? Yes, to a point, but there is no such thing as a total sunblock (98 per cent is the max), and sadly the higher the SPF, the more chemicals you are putting on your skin. Ultimately you should limit your sun exposure (especially between 11am and 3pm, when the sun is most damaging) rather than use a higher SPF sunscreeen.

Fast track If you have dry skin and regularly use a moisturizing foundation, use a lighter moisturizer underneath.

Less is more

less rubbing
less tugging
less cream
less stress

a more *balanced, clear* complexion

What about toner?

My advice is don't bother if you use a rinse-off cleanser and rinse thoroughly. If you use a creamy cleanser, however, you may use toner to remove any residue. But you don't need it.

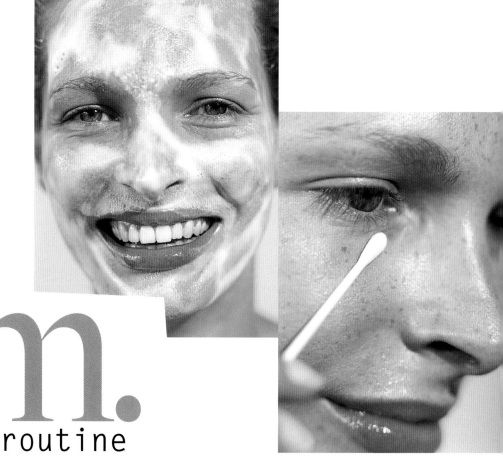

a.m.
routine

Make your morning skincare quick... you've got things to do. But keep it flexible. Look in the mirror before you start each day. Your skin is a living thing. Assess it before you begin.

1 If you cleansed well the night before and there's no shininess by morning, just sweep over a little rosewater to dampen your skin and then moisturize (step 4). If, however, your face is shiny when you wake up, the chances are that it's dirty (dirt and dust adhere to surface oils) so you'll need to cleanse. Warm your cleanser between the palms of your clean hands before applying it to your skin. Whichever type you choose, apply it with your fingertips and massage thoroughly on to your face, around the eyes and over the neck, using circular and then upward movements. The more you massage it in, the better. Remove with water or tissues.

2 Pat your skin dry with a towel if using a rinse-off cleanser, or with a clean tissue if you use a cream cleanser. (If you like using a toner, do so at this point.) Next, assuming you used eye make-up the day before, wipe a cotton pad soaked in a little soothing eye make-up remover lotion over your eyes to help refresh them. Then place the pad you're using over each eye in turn, press on and leave for a few seconds before wiping away. Wipe beneath the eyes with a cotton bud dipped in the same solution. With your eyes free from last night's make-up, today's will look even better.

4 You need just four dots of your moisturizer – one for the forehead, one for each cheek and one for the throat. Pat it gently on to cover your skin rather than smoothing it on. This will help to increase circulation and invigorate your complexion. Then dot a little more moisturizer on the skin around your mouth to minimize any ageing fine lines that may appear there. Finish with a daily layer of sun protection and a little balm over your lips.

Keep looking Some parts of your programme take only a week to show the benefits, others need the full three weeks. Visible changes prove that you are taking very real steps to improve the health and appearance of your skin – and your Nutrition programme is a major part of why it looks so good right now.

5 As a final boost every morning, press your face quite firmly with your palms. This is called 'palming', and it quickly energizes the skin, reduces puffiness and takes away that 'just got up' look that comes increasingly with maturity and poor lymph drainage.

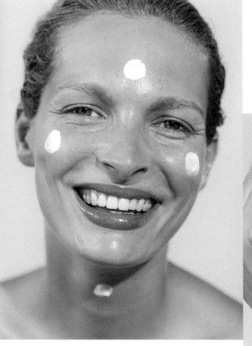

3 Never forget to apply eye cream – it can take off years in seconds. But the way you apply it determines whether you end up with smooth skin or puffy eyes. Dot a tiny amount onto your fingertips and, starting at the outer ends of your laughter lines, lightly pat it onto the skin that covers the orbital bone (you'll feel it under your fingers). Then tap inwards under the eyes, toward the nose. Forget your eyelids – it may slide into the eyes as it warms on the skin.

Don't miss Avoid rinsing with very hot water. It only encourages broken capillaries – the tiniest blood vessels that serve the skin.

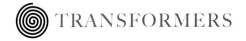

p.m.
routine

Night-time skin beauty is basically all about nourishment: feeding and replenishing your skin with the precious oils and water it needs to stay soft and youthful.

2 Again warming the eye make-up remover lotion, soak a cotton pad with lotion and place over the eye area. Press on and leave for a few seconds before wiping in a down and outward sweep to prevent dragging and rubbing. If you wear waterproof make-up, or use oily remover, follow with a sweep of regular make-up remover because oil can cause watery eyes and puffiness if left on overnight. Finish with a wipe beneath the eyes with moist cotton wool.

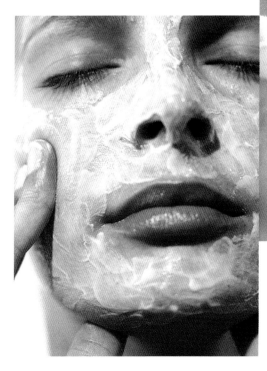

1 Cleansing the day away should be a two-step process: make-up removal followed by all-over facial cleansing. This is because the average cleanser can't cut through the waxes, oils and pigments in make-up to get to the dirt and debris that has built up over the day. Start with a good make-up remover for the face. Warm it first, between your palms, so it will melt the oils and waxes more easily. Then press onto the skin to create a 'suction' effect. This helps to lift make-up off more easily. Use a gently sweeping, outward action and don't rub (to avoid dragging the skin).

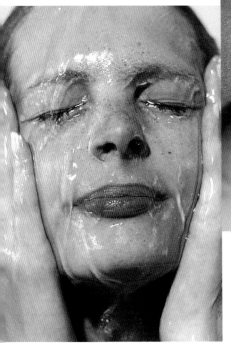

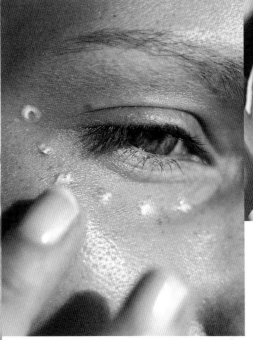

3   Once your make-up's removed, use your usual facial cleanser to give a final cleanse. With both thumbs placed under your chin, use your fingers to massage your cleanser (whether creamy or rinse-off) thoroughly into your skin. It takes no time once you know how.

4   Apply eye cream or gel to the outer area of the orbital bones only – if it's applied too near the eyes at night, the warmth of your skin may make it rub off on the pillow, or slip into your eyes, making them look puffy when you wake.

5   Last thing at night is the perfect moment to spend time massaging in a little facial oil (or serum if you have oily skin). Dry or dehydrated skins will love a blend of carrier oils. Choose three or more from jojoba, vitamin E, evening primrose, avocado and borage oil, mixing together in equal portions, and you have the perfect base for a massage oil that you can use alone or with pure essential oils. Simply close your eyes and combine light, upward sweeping movements and the firm but gentle press-and-release action of the anti-ageing facial massage technique (see page 100), using your fingertips. Follow with either your night cream or serum.

Don't skimp Keep a spare lip balm by your bed (next to the hand cream) and apply last thing before getting into bed.

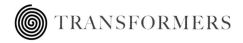

Caring for your eyes

Twenty-two muscles in constant motion mean that your eyes age every time you blink, squint or crinkle up in reaction to sun, wind, smoke, cold, computer screens...or life.

The skin around your eyes is incredibly fine and delicate. It absorbs UV rays more easily than other skin on the body, it has less collagen and elastin, and it loses moisture more quickly too. Not surprisingly, it needs extra care and protection and it's the first place to show wrinkles. But you have the chance to improve everything from now on.

● Sun exposure accounts for 80 per cent of wrinkles, so keep sunglasses in your car and in your bag.
● Like the rest of the body, your eyes need relaxation at frequent intervals: lack of sleep, exercise and fresh air all result in dull, tired eyes.
● A well-balanced diet is vital too. The right foods for eyes include citrus fruits, apricots, green leafy vegetables, carrots, turnips, egg yolk, butter and cheese – all high in vitamin A.
● To keep your eyes clear and sparkling, drink more water and avoid alcohol, late nights and cigarettes.

For sore, tired eyes Soak and chill two camomile tea bags, lie down and place on closed lids for 5 minutes.

To wake up sleepy eyes Place two cotton-wool balls that have been soaked in ice-cold milk over your eyes for 5 minutes.

For puffy eyes This condition is often a result of fluid retention and can be made worse by lying flat at night. So if it looks worse in the morning, try changing your sleeping position. Add an extra pillow to help prevent fluids 'pooling'. And try the sleepy-eyes remedy (above), leaving for 5 minutes and then rinsing with fresh water and patting dry.

For fine lines round your eyes Apply eye cream carefully (see page 89) and wear wrap-around sunglasses with UV100 protection.

Don't miss Make your eyes feel brighter and more alert by pressing for a count of 3 on the pressure point on the bridge of your nose. Feel with your finger for a small dent. Repeat five times.

Looking after your lips

After eyes, your lips are the most vulnerable area in the fight against ageing. It's vital to protect from the drying effects of sun, wind, and central heating or air conditioning.

Lip skin isn't like facial skin: it's thinner and finer, and lacks several of the body's protective substances. As we get older, our lips naturally lose some of their fat and so appear thinner. And gradually, the fragile skin around them becomes prone to fine lines too. Your lips are also a good indication of how you live your life as they're always first to show the signs of fatigue and dehydration.

● Keep on drinking that water.
● Use a moisturizer on the surrounding area too – look for something with skin-saving vitamins A, C and E and a sunscreen with an SPF of 15 minimum to protect against premature ageing.

For dry, cracked lips Apply lip balm regularly, preferably one with SP15 protection. Reapply as often as you can remember throughout the day, rather than waiting for them to get dry. Resist licking your lips – this only makes them drier.

For loose skin Don't pull at it. Make-up artists recommend applying petroleum jelly to soften, and then gently rubbing away at the loose skin with an old toothbrush.

For a conditioning lip mask Mix 5ml of vitamin E oil with one drop of rose essential oil. It gives them an instant, natural shine and helps to condition and protect. Apply at night and leave on.

Change your smile Could it be your teeth that spoil your smile? Professional teeth whitening can take little more than an hour to achieve and makes a dramatic difference to the way you perceive your smile. Then again, you can experiment with lipstick to play up thin lips with gloss, or play down large lips with dark, minimizing colours (see page 160).

Don't miss Dry and cracked lips may indicate a diet high in perservatives and/or intestines not functioning well.

beautifiers

Hopefully you've squeezed your basic skincare regime into your daily programme. Now you need to make time for one (or more) of these fast-acting, weekly beauty treats. They open pores, cleanse and boost circulation, literally bringing your skin to life. Don't miss out.

a quick scrub

FEW BEAUTY TREATMENTS DELIVER SUCH INSTANT RESULTS AS A FACE SCRUB. EXFOLIATION IS THE KEY TO BRIGHTER SKIN BECAUSE IT REMOVES DULL, DEAD CELLS FROM THE SKIN'S SURFACE TO EXPOSE THE FRESHER SKIN BENEATH, AND ENCOURAGES BETTER CELLULAR RENEWAL (ESSENTIAL FOR YOUNGER-LOOKING SKIN IN 21 DAYS).

It takes less time than you'd think. You can exfoliate your face in under a minute so add it to your regime – after cleansing and before your moisturizer.

But remember that golden skincare rule: less is more. While young skin (15–35 years) is thick, supple and resilient, older skin (35 years plus) is thinner and more susceptible to external damage. And while sloughing off those dead skin cells helps to make skin look brighter and clearer at any age, experts now warn against making fine skin thinner still because that can accelerate the effects of environmental ageing.

You can exfoliate your skin using a grainy scrub (containing artificial beads or natural grains), a buffing cloth, or a chemical exfoliant, such as an AHA (alphahydroxy acid) cream or enzyme cream. Only by understanding your own skin better (see page 83) will you know what suits it. Whichever type of scrub you choose, exfoliate just once a week (or every other week if you have sensitive skin), and for no longer than a minute.

Concentrate scrubs around oilier, congested areas, such as the nose, chin and forehead. Never use a grainy scrub on the delicate skin around your eyes and moisturize straightaway.

Grainy scrubs contain tiny particles which, when massaged into the skin, help to lift out dirt and impurities and rub off dead skin cells. Choose carefully: natural walnut and apricot grains, cut from the kernel, often have sharp edges that may scratch the skin's surface. Opt for artificial, perfectly rounded, spherical beads that are gentler on your skin.

You can try out the effect of a facial scrub by adding a little sugar, salt or oatmeal to your usual cleanser. Dampen your face, massage as usual and then rinse thoroughly with clean water. Use a face cloth or muslin to remove tiny traces from around the nose.

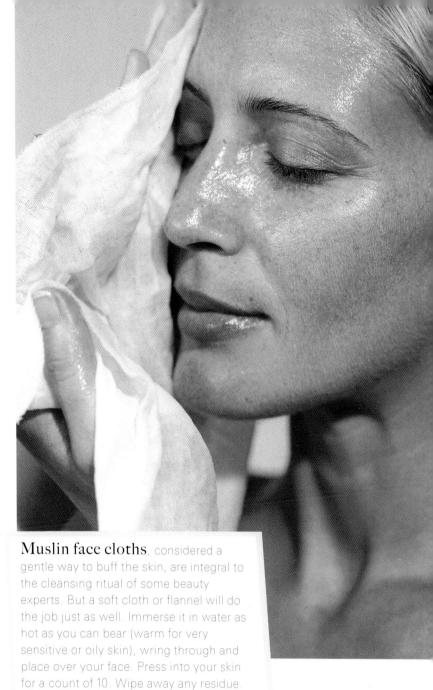

2 fruity exfoliating treatments To make at home

Lemon & sugar scrub

Oily and combination skin. Put a handful of brown sugar in a small bowl and squeeze in the juice of half a lemon. Mix together and massage gently on to your skin, over the forehead, cheeks, nose, chin, throat and chest. Wipe off with a damp muslin cloth. Rinse thoroughly with plenty of fresh, warm water. Pat your skin dry.

Peachy scrub

Normal to dry skin. Pulp one large peach and mix together with one dessertspoon of finely ground oatmeal (not flakes). Massage over your face, paying particular attention to any congested areas, and rinse off with warm water.

Exfoliating creams and lotions

often contain enzymes or AHAs. Enzyme exfoliators are generally based on naturally occurring enzymes, such as papain from papaya, or bromelian, the enzyme found in pineapple. Left on the skin for just a few minutes, these gentle but active substances work by dissolving dead skin cells, leaving skin brighter and smoother. AHA creams (see page 112) work by actually loosening dead skin. Research shows that AHAs can also help your skin reinforce its own barrier function and its ability to renew itself. However, they have also been found to trigger skin problems in some people, especially those who have delicate or sensitive skin.

Muslin face cloths, considered a

gentle way to buff the skin, are integral to the cleansing ritual of some beauty experts. But a soft cloth or flannel will do the job just as well. Immerse it in water as hot as you can bear (warm for very sensitive or oily skin), wring through and place over your face. Press into your skin for a count of 10. Wipe away any residue. Repeat two or three times if necessary

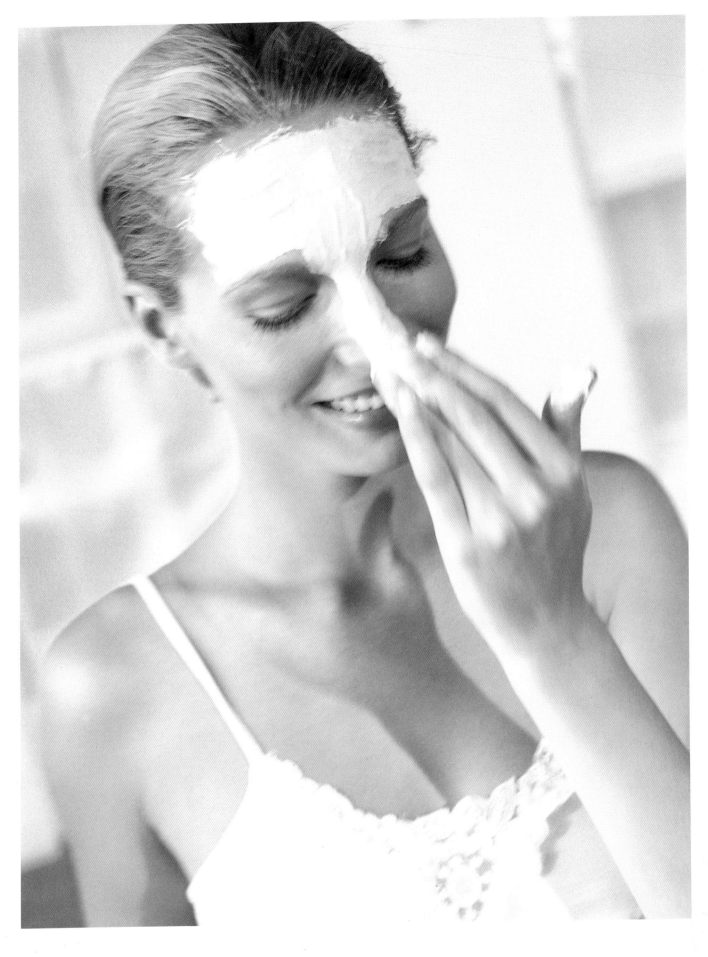

time for a mask

IF THERE'S ONE PRODUCT WELL WORTH SQUEEZING INTO YOUR WEEKLY SKINCARE PROGRAMME, IT'S A FACE MASK. AND THERE'S ONE TO SUIT EVERY SKIN TYPE. APPLY TO CLEAN SKIN, LEAVE ON FOR THE TIME STATED ON THE PACK – ANYWHERE BETWEEN 1 AND 10 MINUTES – NO LONGER OR YOU MAY IRRITATE YOUR SKIN. WASH, PEEL OR TISSUE OFF, DEPENDING ON THE TYPE, AND THEN FOLLOW UP WITH YOUR USUAL MOISTURIZER.

Skincare experts now believe in the power of layering products on top of each other. The theory (even evidence) is that in this way each product can enhance the action of the others, so your skin gets precisely what it needs at any given time. Few skins, for example, are oily or dry all over – you get patchy zones of dehydration with oily skin, or dry skin with an oily T-zone. By layering different face masks, your skin can take what it needs. But best of all, masks make you feel positively spoilt and decadent, and heaven knows we all like a bit of that every now and then.

Many masks contain flower or herbal extracts and plant oils to improve the skin's appearance. Choose one or more of these basic mask types.

Deep-cleansing masks help to absorb excess oils and impurities, and cleanse pores deep down. They include clay, tar and seaweed extracts – often scented with menthol and camphor – to give that astringent element and the traditional dry, on-the-verge-of-cracking feel and appearance. Never leave on for longer than stated on the pack as they can be extremely stimulating. These are ideal for any skin type that needs deep cleansing, especially oily or combination skin that is especially prone to blocked pores from excess sebum and dirt.

Peel-off masks help to eliminate the dead skin cells that make your complexion look dull and dirty, so they are great for both dry and oily skin. They are usually gel-like and dry in minutes. Wait the recommended time before peeling off otherwise they can be hard to remove.

Exfoliating masks If blackheads and congestion are the problem, exfoliating masks, which work rather like a face scrub, are better still. Some may include enzymes that work by dissolving surface dead skin cells. These are gentler than they might sound so give them a try.

Moisturizing masks are thick and creamy and incorporate lots of superior moisturizing ingredients, such as hyaluronic acid, along with ingredients to stimulate circulation. They rarely dry on the skin and are used more to plump, soften and iron out signs of ageing and tiredness. Needless to say they're great for dry and dehydrated skin. And remember that even oily skin can be dehydrated, because it's water that's in short supply here, not oil – but you'd probably want to leave them off the T-zone.

Revitalizing masks are quickie, emergency pick-me-ups that refresh and give radiance. Some plump up to counteract dehydration, a few exfoliate too, but most contain menthol, camphor or some other cooling, skin-tightening ingredient to boost the circulation, make skin feel tingly and give it a healthy glow by stimulating blood capillaries. If your skin frequently looks tired, you'll want one of these. They provide an excellent pep-up any time you need it, especially after a long day or before a party, but other than that do little to cleanse or condition the skin. Avoid if you have especially sensitive skin.

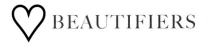
close your eyes and steam

STEAMING IS BENEFICIAL FOR ALL SKIN TYPES, BUT IT CAN BE QUITE STIMULATING SO STICK TO JUST ONCE A WEEK, EITHER AS A BEAUTIFIER DURING YOUR PM REGIME OR DURING YOUR RELAXING FACIAL BOOSTER. FOR DRY, MATURE OR SENSITIVE SKINS, THE MOISTURE HELPS TO PLUMP UP DEHYDRATED SKIN CELLS GENTLY, WHILE FOR OILY AND COMBINATION SKINS THE HEAT WARMS AND SOFTENS BLACKHEADS (THOSE PLUGS OF SEBUM AND DIRT THAT ARE THE MAIN CAUSE OF SPOTS).

1 Fill a large bowl with hot water that has boiled and stood for 5 minutes (a gentle heat is all that is needed). Add either a handful of herbs or a few drops of the appropriate essential or carrier oil (see below and page 220). The oil forms tiny droplets that are easily absorbed by the skin as you steam.

2 Place a medium-sized towel over your head and neck and lean forward over the bowl.

3 Close your eyes, and lower the towel at the front so that it forms a tent and allows the steam vapour to work on your face for up to 3 minutes.

4 Pat your skin dry with a clean towel and then apply your usual moisturizer.

Normal to dry skin Lavender and camomile essential oils

Normal to oily skin A few sprigs of fresh mint and a curl of lemon peel

Dry skin Evening primrose oil or jojoba carrier oil

Hot towel technique

To relax your skin Fill a basin with hot water and dip in a clean flannel or muslin face-cloth. Wring through and, while still hot, wipe over specific areas of the skin. Heat draws out impurities, but many devotees claim that it can stimulate certain muscle groups to minimize fine lines and wrinkles.

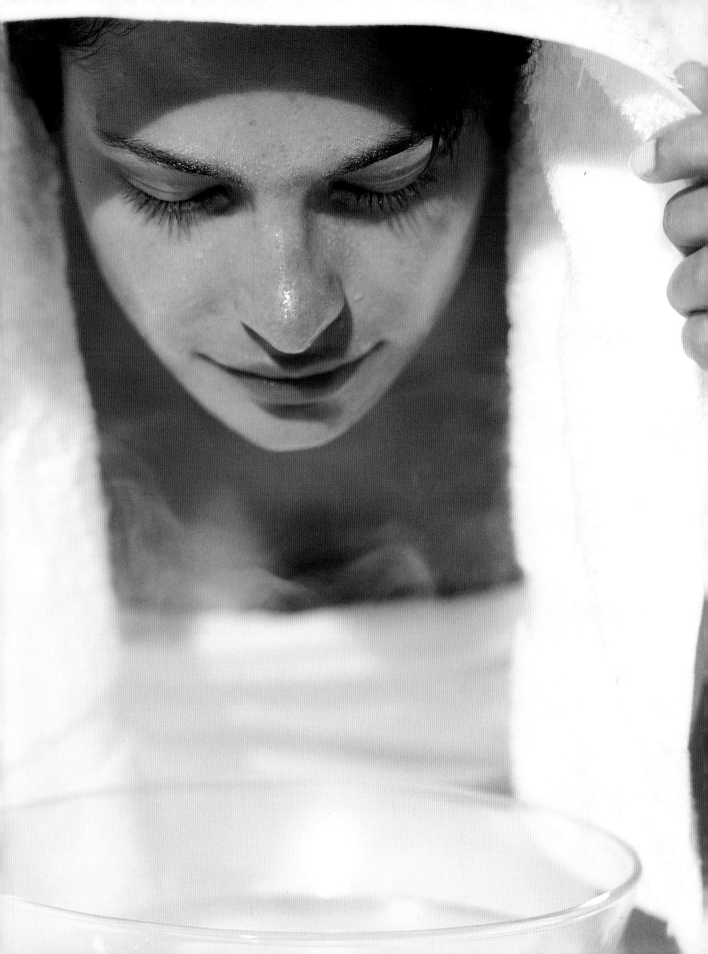

boosters

Relaxing or uplifting, smoothing or softening...anytime you have the time, make space for one of these dramatic skin boosters. They take a little more effort than your beautifiers but, although you may only do them once in these 21 days, I guarantee you'll feel the difference.

anti-ageing facial massage

A QUICK PRESSURE-POINT FACIAL MASSAGE RELIEVES TENSION AND AIDS LYMPHATIC DRAINAGE, GIVING AN INSTANT LIFT AND A YOUTHFUL LOOK TO YOUR FACE. MASTER THIS TECHNIQUE OVER THE NEXT 21 DAYS SO THAT YOU CAN BOOST THE TONE AND TEXTURE OF YOUR COMPLEXION WHENEVER NEEDED. THIS WAY YOU CAN INCORPORATE DIFFERENT MASSAGE STEPS WHILE YOU APPLY YOUR DAILY MOISTURIZER (A,B,D & E) OR EYECARE (B & C) OR ON BARE SKIN IN THE MIDDLE OF THE EVENING WITH EITHER A NOURISHING FACIAL OIL, NIGHT CREAM OR SKIN SERUM.

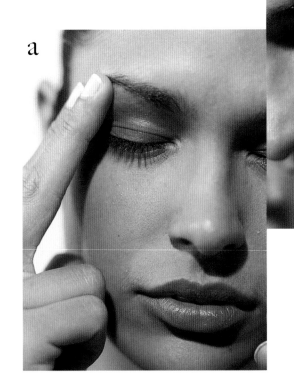

b

a

To smooth forehead Start by applying gentle pressure at the bridge of your nose with the tips of each index and middle finger and then release. Glide up to the inner ends of your eyebrows to press and release, then over your brows to the outer ends to press and release again, and finally to your temples. Repeat the sequence twice.

To lift eyes Place three fingers just under your brows, press and release. Repeat on the brow, and twice up to the hairline.

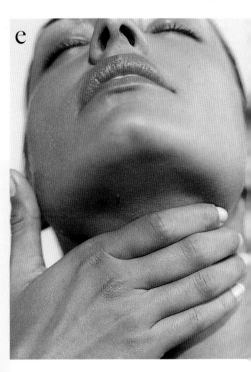

To lift throat

Keep your fingers together as you use upward, sweeping movements with alternate fingers and palms, working from the clavicle bone up the neck to your jawline. Repeat the sequence twice.

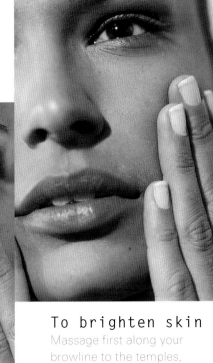

To brighten skin

Massage first along your browline to the temples, using your fingertips in tiny, light, sweeping, upward movements, and then across the forehead to the temples Next massage across your lower face, working gently under your eyes, then from the sides of your nostrils and finally from your chin out toward your ears. Repeat the whole sequence twice.

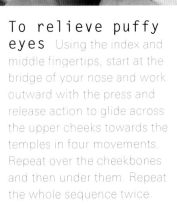

To relieve puffy eyes

Using the index and middle fingertips, start at the bridge of your nose and work outward with the press and release action to glide across the upper cheeks towards the temples in four movements. Repeat over the cheekbones and then under them. Repeat the whole sequence twice.

Facial oils These are only recommended for those with dry or mature skins. Try two drops of pure rose essential oil with two drops of neroli essential oil in 10ml (1 tbsp) of jojoba carrier oil for a mix with a well-loved smell. Or blend 3ml of wheatgerm carrier oil with one drop of pure rose essential oil. Or simply use almond carrier oil on its own. Store mixtures in a small, dark bottle – oils are degraded by light – and shake well before use. (Look for rose otto, derived by steam distillation, rather than rose absolute, derived by chemical extraction.)

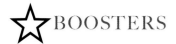

relaxing facial

TREAT YOURSELF TO A HOME FACIAL EACH WEEK. IT DOESN'T HAVE TO BE LABOURED –
A SIMPLE CLEANSE, STEAM, SCRUB, SPRITZ, MASK AND MASSAGE WILL DO THE TRICK.
DON'T RUB, POKE OR SQUEEZE ANYTHING. (USE A DEEP-CLEANSING MASK IF YOU FEEL
THE NEED.) TAKE A LITTLE EXTRA TIME TO MASSAGE IN EACH PRODUCT, LAYER BY
LAYER. TRY COMBINING A FEW OF YOUR NEW MASSAGE TECHNIQUES (SEE THE PREVIOUS
PAGE) TO MAKE IT ALL THE MORE PLEASURABLE. PAT YOUR SKIN DRY BETWEEN EACH STEP
WITH FRESH, CLEAN TISSUES (JUST AS A BEAUTY THERAPIST WOULD). AND TURN THE
WHOLE THING INTO A RITUALISTIC TREAT – MUCH LIKE A SALON FACIAL.

Use this session as a measure of your skin's progress, monitoring its improvement at the end of each seven days, and helping you to get to know it better with every step of the programme. Before you start, ensure you have a warm, cosy room, everything you need to hand, hair pulled back out of the way, and clothing (i.e. a bathrobe) that can be splashed or removed easily.

1 Begin by cleansing your skin. Warm the cleanser between the palms of your hands and then massage into your skin with firm, circular movements. If it's a creamy cleanser, take a clean tissue, make a tiny slit in the middle of it, and place this over your nose, pressing the tissue onto your skin to increase absorption and then finally wipe off the remaining cream. If you use a rinse-off cleanser, remember to give your face several (no less than three) splashes of clean water, and remove any final residue of cleanser with a damp muslin face-cloth or flannel.

2 Try a little light steam unless you have very dry skin. Fill a bowl with hot water, and add a few fresh herbs from the garden, such as lavender, basil and rosemary. Or use one drop of each of the related essential oils. With a medium-sized towel draped over your head and the bowl in the usual way, breathe in deeply (also great if you have sinus problems) and stay like this for up to 3 minutes, depending on how sensitive your skin is and how comfortable you are.

3 Gently exfoliate to buff away any remaining dead skin cells that have become loose after cleansing and steaming, making sure your skin still feels damp before you begin and focusing on areas of congestion. Rinse thoroughly with warm water. If appropriate, use a muslin face-cloth (or soft flannel) to ensure that you've removed any remaining grains from around the nose, in the hairline and under the chin.

4 A facial spritzer is a great pick-me-up for your skin at this moment. Many beauty therapists use toning sprays between cleansers and masks. Make your own inexpensive one from pure rosewater – it's suitable for all skin types. Either spritz or apply with cotton-wool pads.

5 Apply a face mask. Choose one depending on how your skin looks and feels (see page 97). Close your eyes and lie back for the specified time, anything up to 10 minutes. Remove, using muslin (or flannel) to get the last traces off your skin.

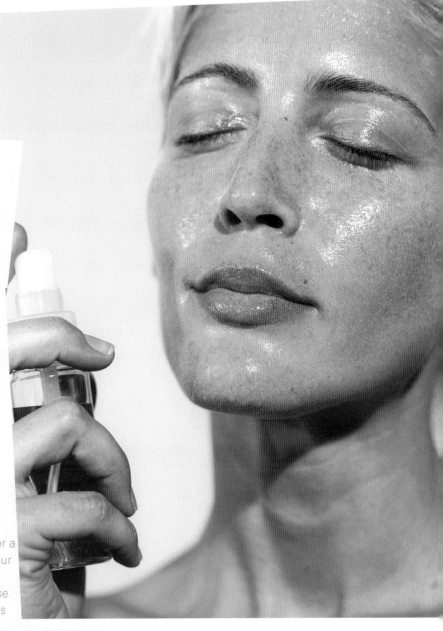

6 Massage your skin, using a facial-oil mix for dry/mature skin (see page 101) or a lighter serum. Place the fingertips of your index, middle and ring fingers on your eyebrows, press slowly, and then release. Repeat twice. Now move your fingertips to the lower socket area (just under the eyes) and again, with a light and slow action, press and release three times. Sweep your fingertips up to the centre of your forehead, facing each other, and then press outwards toward the temples on either side. Continue to press along the hairline, past the cheekbones, pinching the earlobes, and along the jawline until your fingertips finally meet at the chin. Blot off any excess oil or serum with a clean tissue,

7 For a finishing touch, apply your day moisturizer, night cream or anti-ageing treatment, depending on your skin's needs. Take a little extra time to massage the cream in so that the process feels more indulgent.

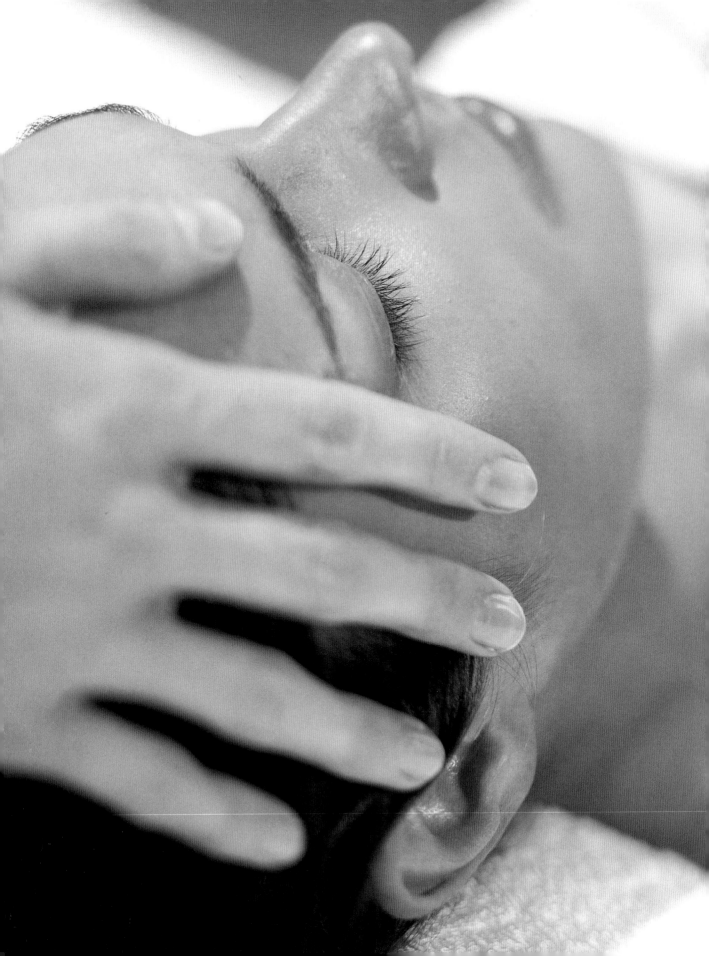

what about a salon facial?

HAVING A FACIAL ISN'T JUST ABOUT LAYERS OF CREAMS AND MASKS TO PLUMP UP AND SOFTEN YOUR SKIN, THOUGH THERE'S NO DENYING THAT'S PART OF THE ALLURE. THE MOST BENEFICIAL THING ABOUT HAVING A SALON FACIAL – OR GIVING YOURSELF ONE AT HOME – IS THAT YOU'RE TAKING THE TIME OUT SOLELY FOR YOU. A MIND/BODY THING, THE EXPERIENCE GOES WAY BEYOND SKIN DEEP, AND CAN FEEL WONDERFULLY RESTORATIVE IF IT'S DONE DURING THE DAY (SAY A WEEKDAY LUNCHTIME) OR IN THE EARLY EVENING. AND YOU MAY BE SURPRISED TO FIND HOW LONG THE FEEL-GOOD FACTOR LASTS – AT LEAST SEVEN DAYS, I'D SAY.

A professional salon facial has the great benefit of treating your skin to one entire product range. And that's great at a time when, perhaps, you feel you're stuck in a rut with a tired old skincare regime and want to try something new. So take an hour of your time to reinforce your beauty programme with one of the range of procedures on offer.

Some treatments provide a high-quality, high-skill alternative to what you can achieve at home – and I guarantee that your own skincare rituals will improve ten-fold following a professional facial. Others use various different forms of electrotherapy to help stimulate the facial muscles, improving muscle tone and skin elasticity, albeit temporarily. These are great as a one-off for a special occasion or as a course of treatments to give your skin a real boost.

Massage and plant-based products, including homeopathic ampoules and essential oils, feature widely in the more low-tech treatments to leave your skin looking and feeling really fabulous. Some, based on holistic principles, offer a deep-focus mind/body treatment that aims to re-balance and re-harmonize the skin and body and leaves you feeling calm and soothed from head to toe.

If you're going professional

● Speak up. Be confident enough to say if you are not happy about something, whether it is the temperature of the room, the music that's playing or some part of the facial that you don't like. It's your time and your money – don't waste either.

● Every professional facial should have a mini-consultation first, to check that you have no contra-indications. Tell the therapist if you are pregnant, have a medical condition (epilepsy or a pacemaker are clear contra-indications for electrotherapy treatments) or if you are already using a daily skin treatment such as the acne/anti-ageing vitamin A cream Retinova (known as Retin-A in the USA).

● Expect to remove your shoes and the top half of your clothing. So avoid wearing a dress – or socks with holes. You will also be asked to remove your jewellery. Some facials may leave oil around your hairline – so it's best to check ahead if you intend to go straight out in the evening.

● Ideally don't re-apply make-up after a facial. Arrange for an afternoon/early evening appointment and then head home for your favourite relaxation exercises (see chapter 7) and your blissful bedtime ritual (see page 124).

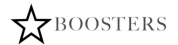

zone in on your skin

HOLISTIC SKINCARE EXPERTS BELIEVE EVERY LIFE EVENT IS WRITTEN ON YOUR FACE. USING FACE MAPPING, ONE OF TRADITIONAL CHINESE MEDICINE'S ANCIENT ARTS, THEY STUDY THE SKIN IN DIFFERENT ZONES OF THE FACE FOR INDICATIONS OF HEALTH AND WELLBEING, OFTEN PICKING UP SLIGHT IMBALANCES IN THE BODY, WHICH THEY TREAT WITH REFLEXOLOGY, OR MANUAL PRESSURE DESIGNED TO PROMOTE AN INTERNAL FLOW OF ENERGY THAT HELPS STIMULATE THE NATURAL PROCESSES OF SELF-HEALING. WORK THE ZONES FOR AT LEAST 15 MINUTES AS OFTEN AS YOU CAN (DAILY IF POSSIBLE), AND BY WEEK THREE YOU SHOULD SEE AN IMPROVEMENT IN YOUR SKIN AND OVERALL HEALTH.

Reflexologists believe each part of the body relates to a corresponding area on the face as well as on the feet (and even the hands), and that pressure on these 'reflex zones' can release the minor tensions that may be blocking the internal flow of energy within the related body part. Reflexology will also eliminate waste matter that may have accumulated in the body because of ill health or stress (a major factor in as much as 80 per cent of all illnesses).

The map opposite shows the reflex zones in the face. Read the face-map key (right) and you find, for example, that if the skin on your chin often gets quite congested with blackheads, it may result either from tensions in the pancreas (a vital organ of cleansing) or in the reproductive organs (typically, in this case blackheads appear at either side of the mouth and may well be linked to your monthly cycle). And if the skin around your eyes appears darker, you may have kidney problems.

During these 21 days, concentrate your attention particularly on zones where you currently have a problem. Feel the skin on your face with your fingertips, gently pressing as you go. You should soon discover 'dents', areas where your fingers seem to sink further into the skin. Press at those points and hold for a count of five (repeating between five and ten times).

How to read your face

Face mapping and reflexology are an effective way to diagnose and treat minor conditions, but always consult your health practitioner if you have grounds for serious concern.

Zone 1 This area reflects the health of the intestines. Spots and congestion may mean the colon is congested or being cleansed. Redness here may mean too much salt, red meat or dairy foods are being consumed (all of which are stimulating to the body). If the skin looks white, cut back on sugar and caffeine.

Zone 2 The liver is stimulated here. Tension or imbalance in this area is reflected in breakouts and premature wrinkles. Cut back on alcohol and preservatives.

Zones 3 & 4 These areas reflect conditions in the kidneys (near the inner corners of the eyes) and the lungs (on the cheeks). Skin irritations or congestion around the cheeks or sides of the nose are linked to too much dairy in the diet.

Zone 5 The end of the nose relates to the heart. Redness, broken capillaries or swelling may reveal high blood pressure and a cardiovascular system under stress.

Zones 6, 7 & 8 The chin area forms the end of the T-zone and is the site of an abundance of sebaceous glands. In Chinese diagnosis, breakouts here relate to the reproductive organs and hormonal fluctuation. The position of spots during menstruation is said to indicate from which side a woman is ovulating.

Zone 9 Pressure on the neck and thyroid area can boost your metabolism. Often neglected in skincare rituals, dry, crepey necks are common because there are few sebaceous glands in the neck.

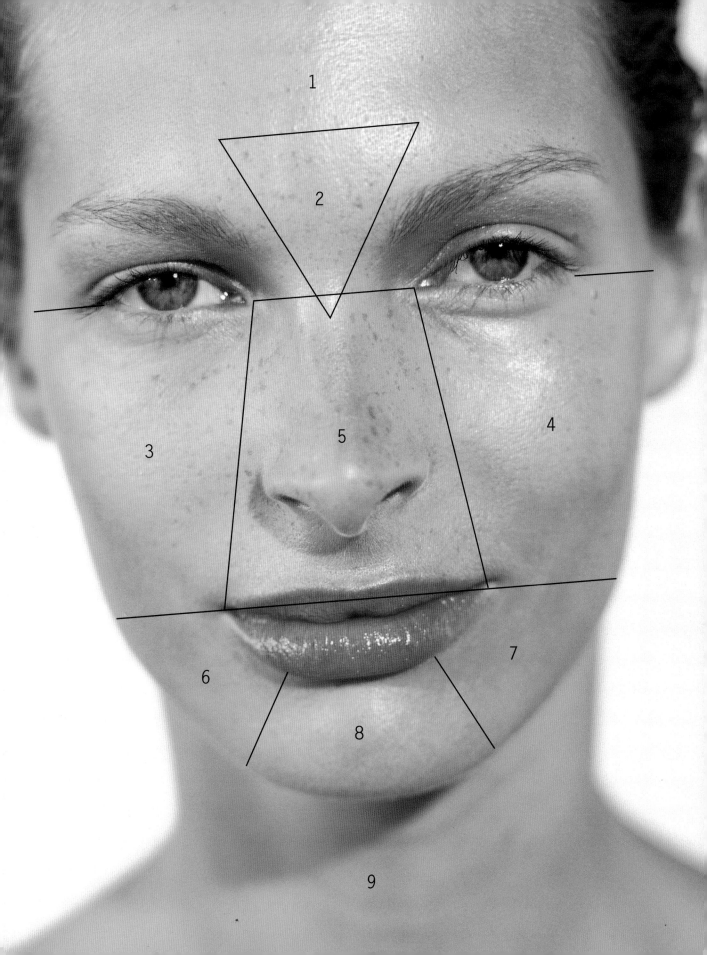

Replace every cup of coffee or tea you drink with a cup of hot water. It's refreshing and after the first week you'll notice a difference in your skin.

Go gently Place your thumbs on your chin before massaging in a facial exfoliator. This will give you a gentler action which is less likely to irritate the skin.

Misting It's something every woman should do. Carry a bottle and spray your face throughout the day: first thing, under moisturizer to encourage skin to absorb more moisture, over your morning make-up to seal it, and then to freshen it up at the end of the day. Keep a bottle in your handbag, on your bedside table and on your desk; and don't fly without it.

Use a protective day cream every day Choose one that's high in antioxidants and with an SPF15 UV protection, whether it's cloudy or sunny, to protect skin from the free radicals that cause wrinkles.

After cleansing Splash your skin up to 30 times with fresh warm water or use a muslin cloth or soft flannel to stimulate the skin before moisturizing.

Nourish your neck Always use a separate cream or serum on your chest. Gravity is constantly pulling down, there are no muscles as such to support the bust and it loses elasticity very quickly.

To reduce puffiness Take the heat out of skin by wrapping a small ice-cube in a hanky and gliding it out from the inside corner of the nose (near the eye) to the ear and down that side of the face to just under the jaw. Repeat on both sides.

Bump up your vitamin C It's essential for collagen production, which keeps skin soft and supple, and it isn't stored in the body so take a supplement.

Tiny red thread veins? Found more commonly on the cheeks and nose of those with fair skin, they are caused by exposure to heat, cold or wind. So treat your skin gently. Avoid using very hot water, and protect your skin in extreme temperatures. Wear a moisturizer daily, and an SPF 15 sunscreen to prevent more damage.

If your skin feels very dry Increase your water intake. Remember your aim is to drink 2 litres (3 ½pt) of mineral water a day.

Shiny T-zone? Leave moisturizer off the area for a few days (many contain mineral oil which tends to clog the pores). Then, after a week, to keep things in check, try a T-zone control gel that contains powder particles to absorb oil.

Spots and blackheads Just around your hairline and cheeks? You may be using cosmetics that block your pores. Use only 'non-comedogenic' cosmetics (comedones = blackheads). Around your nose and chin? Your pores may be getting clogged with sebum. Steam and exfoliate once a week.

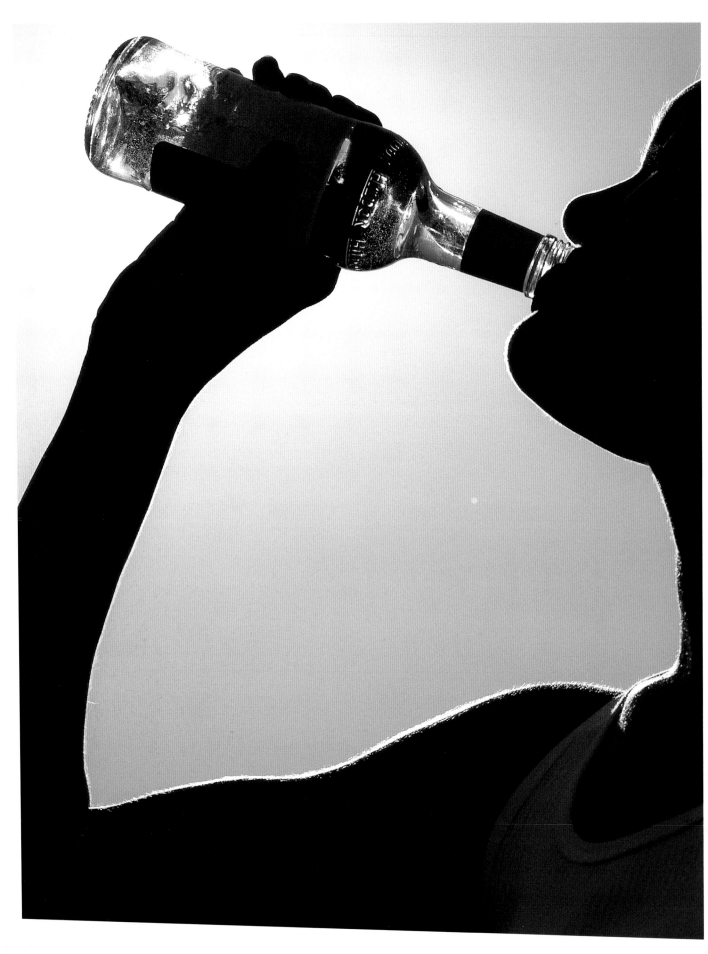

keeping it going

Seek balance

You can't avoid wrinkles, but try to keep your face from tension and worry. An expressive face lines faster according to cosmetic surgeons, which is fine if you have lots of positive-looking laughter lines. But a worried expression increases wrinkles around the forehead, the bridge of the nose and the mouth, which can take on a downward turn, and that makes you look unhappy – even when you aren't! So, with wrinkles inevitable, keep up all those de-stressing techniques in chapter 7.

Check your eyes

Aim to keep your eyes looking well rested and well nurtured. Eyes are truly the windows to the soul – and instant indicators of our health. See how they sparkle now, making the whites positively luminescent. Lack of sleep, a poorly balanced diet and anxiety quickly dim that brightness.

Choose a better path

Stop smoking It causes premature lines around the eyes and lips. Smoke also restricts oxygen and nutrient supply to the skin, depleting the vitamin C vital for collagen production.

Cut back on alcohol Red wine in moderation can benefit your health but constantly finishing the bottle won't. Alcohol is sugar, it also dehydrates and dilates blood capillaries.

Change your diet forever Maintain that increase in 'coloured' fruit and vegetables – all high in the antioxidants which protect from ageing – and cut right down on junk food.

Avoid margarine, fried foods and sugar Margarine, a hydrogenated fat, blocks the body's ability to use skin-boosting EFAs (see page 40). Fried foods clog the skin's pores. And sugar interferes with the absorption of skin-enhancing minerals such as zinc, magnesium and calcium.

Cut down on caffeine It inhibits the absorption of vitamins and minerals.

Bump up on supplements Evening primrose oil contains gamma-linolenic acid (GLA), an essential fatty acid that helps to boost the moisture content of your skin.

Drink more water The more you can keep within your skin the better.

Limit your sun exposure Now you know that sun alone is responsible for around 80 per cent of skin ageing, protect your skin from UV rays, whether it's cloudy or sunny. Let your body be in the sun, sure, but keep your face out. If you like a tanned face, fake it. If you wear foundation, good. It acts as a great daily sunblock because the tiny powder particles are light reflecting and made from the same material (either zinc oxide or titanium dioxide) as the physical sunscreen in your suncream. By protecting your skin daily with sunscreen, you are helping your skin to repair and regenerate itself naturally.

Stay aware

You know what you put into your body reflects on the outside. But all kinds of hormonal imbalances can cause skin problems too. Give your body a regular MOT to ensure that you're as healthy as you can be and practise face mapping to recognize the way your body feels by looking at your face.

Look for anti-agers in your creams and lotions

Alpha hydroxy acids (AHAs) loosen dead skin so that it sheds to reveal a fresher, smoother complexion. Research shows that AHAs can also help your skin retain more moisture and speed up cell renewal. An AHA product can't make skin more taut or get rid of wrinkles, but it can make it look clearer and more radiant instantly. Citric, glycolic, lactic and malic acids are all examples of AHAs. (Some AHAs have been known to trigger skin problems in those with fair or sensitive skin.)

Enzymes are natural proteins and the latest thing in skincare technology. Skin naturally contains 'good' and 'bad' enzymes. By harnessing beneficial enzymes and stopping production of harmful ones, in theory skin is better able to protect itself.

Retinol (or retinyl) is the collective term for vitamin A derivatives. They help reduce the appearance of age spots and fine lines, and smooth the skin's surface, but their long-term effect is still unknown.

Antioxidants are mostly vitamins – betacarotene (the precursor of vitamin A), C and E, plus zinc, and a few plants (see below). Including them in your diet or as supplements gives the best natural protection from the ageing effects of free-radical damage (see page 34). They are also used in skin and suncare products for additional environmental protection. *Echinacea*, known for its ability to boost the immune system, helps to stimulate cellular repair and is an anti-inflammatory. *Ginkgo biloba* has powerful antioxidant properties. Studies also show that ginkgo leaves have a moisturizing effect, are anti-inflammatory and stimulate the microcirculation. *Green tea* is another powerful antioxidant, inhibiting the release of free radicals in skin. Research shows it can reduce numbers of sunburn cells produced under UV light by up to 67 per cent. *Lycopene* is an antioxidant and a very powerful free-radical scavenger. It's found in tomatoes (cooking them releases it), pink grapefruit, red grapes and watermelon. A deficiency is now associated with acne and dermatitis.

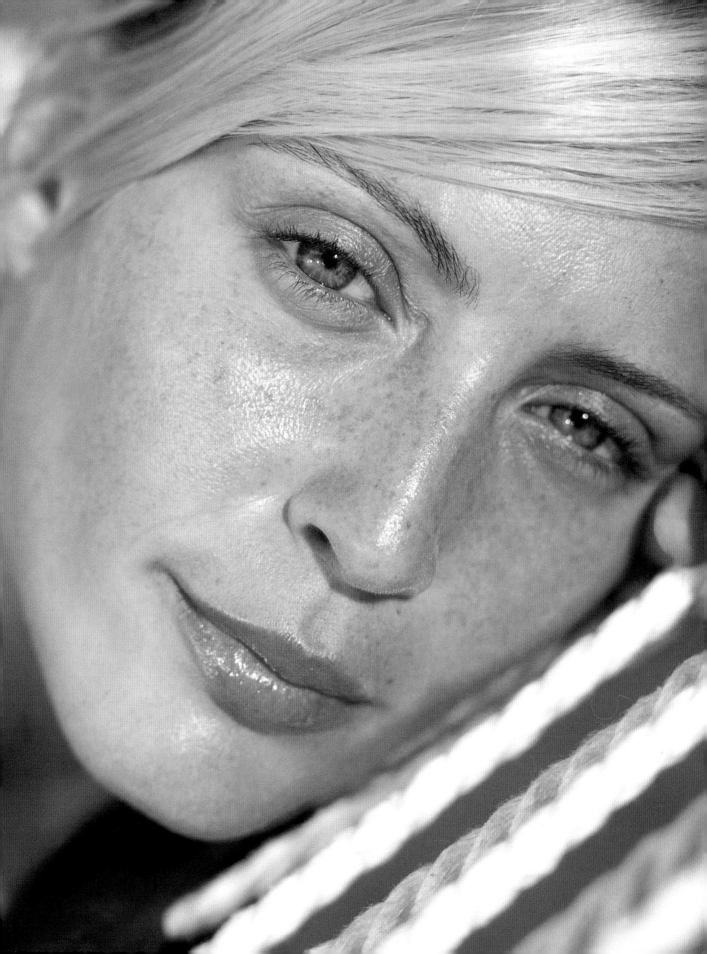

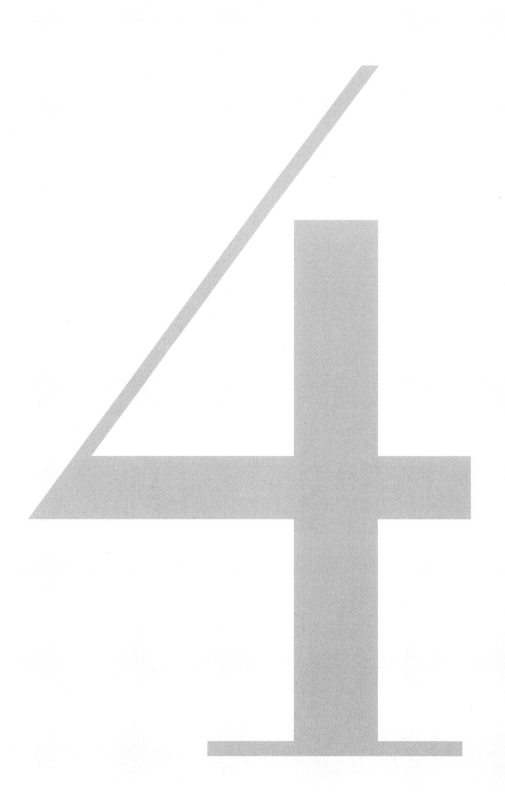

21 DAYS TO BODY CONFIDENCE

Learning to appreciate your body a little more every day - its strength, suppleness and total uniqueness - is the path to loving yourself more.

Your bodycare programme

This is a better-body care regime. It includes all the things you might have remembered to do occasionally - spurred on by a weekend away at a spa or after joining a gym (turning up for a month but then never again). It's not dramatic or life changing - but it is effective. It will rev up your skin tone and remove the lumps and bumps caused by poor micro-circulation, so ultimately your body looks brighter and feels a lot smoother.

REMEMBER YOUR BODY IS AFFECTED BY EVERYTHING YOU DO AND THE WAY YOU FEEL - AND IT SHOWS.

Listening in As you use this more informed daily regime, changing lifelong health and beauty bodycare patterns over the next 21 days, you will naturally become more aware of your body. Look at it objectively. Ask yourself how you're feeling, what you need right now. Listen to your body. You've already assessed it from a fitness point of view. This is the icing – how your body looks and feels. There are treatments here that can, done regularly, work significant improvements. See how, boosted by the achievements in your Fitness and Nutrition programmes, you are taking real steps towards a healthier, happier future.

But I hate the way I look Hating your cellulite or saggy thighs means you're always down on yourself. Look in the mirror regularly and focus on the parts of your body you do like – perhaps you have enviably long legs, or neat ankles, or graceful hands, or an elegant neck, or a pretty smile. These are the things that people will notice about you on meeting! See the positive in all things. Until you accept yourself, no amount of commitment to these programmes is going help you look or feel better about yourself from within.

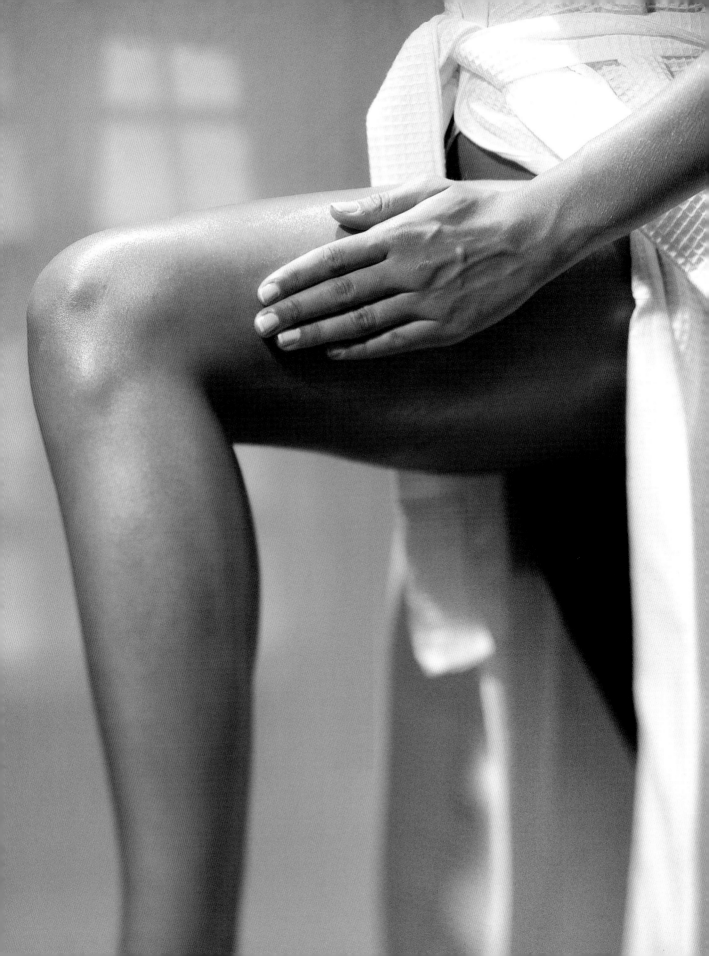

What you do in these 21 days

if you're 20-35...

Your skin is still stretchy, supple and quick to heal. Although body skin is thicker than facial skin, if you sunbathed during your teens and twenties, UV light will have reduced its elasticity, especially on bony areas such as the chest and the hands, leading to coarser skin and even a few premature fine lines. If you've given birth, your body image may well have changed – for better or worse. Take the positive stance – you've won some life scars, be they stretch marks, Caesarean scar or a baby belly. Lavish attention on yourself from now on.

● Protect your hands and chest daily from UV light as you do your face. Remember: damage prevention at this age is your most important anti-ageing skincare tactic.
● Incorporate beautifying treatments such as a body scrub, body wrap and fake tan once a week, along with a regular pedicure and manicure.
● Keep on drinking that water.

...or 35-50

Unless you've been exercising regularly, it is likely your body has been losing muscle tone and gaining body fat. Cellulite may be more pronounced due to poor lymphatic drainage and a higher level of toxins due to your busy lifestyle. But it's not too late to improve.

● Buff that body back into shape. Regular exfoliation, whether with dry body-brushing or a scrub, will boost circulation, making your skin more toned and clear.
● Moisturize twice daily. Make it a new rule after washing. Pamper problem areas with moisturizing creams and potions, and indulge in a few weekly detox treatments using mud and seaweed.
● Keep your hands and chest out of the sun – age spots may become more noticeable now. Look for anti-ageing, vitamin-rich, skin- smoothing creams that help to reduce their appearance. Keep up the fake tan instead.
● Try to reduce any major stresses and keep moving.

... or 50 and over

Hormonal changes mean that your skin may well feel drier and look less elastic – especially around the throat, the chest and the backs of your arms and hands.

● Scrub your skin regularly
● Moisturize that body. Pamper your skin with layers of creams and lotions to boost your natural moisture levels.
● Keep on protecting your skin from the sun. It's never too late to slow down the signs of ageing – skin is constantly renewing, albeit at a slower rate.
● Plump up your skin from within by eating well (losing vast quantities of weight in one go is very ageing from now on).
● Regular exercise at a moderate pace combined with a sensible diet is still the most effective body regime.

What you'll achieve

Confidence You'll feel empowered to live a full life, free from the niggling aches and pains that we associate with getting older – sensations that are often more lifestyle-led than age-determined. It's all too easy to lose confidence in yourself when Western society sets an ideal of physical perfection that's hard to live up to. But it's not just a Western thing: being thin in the Third World through poverty is just as undesirable as it is to be obese in the West through lack of willpower. The fact is neither extreme is healthy. And a healthy body – whatever its size – is what matters. By giving your body everything it needs to be strong, healthy and resilient (and that includes good nutrition and regular exercise), you boost your confidence immeasurably.

Focus You will gain the sort of focus you may have known when pregnant or seen in friends who were pregnant. It's a trust in the nurturing, protecting power of the body. Really pampering yourself – and exercising and eating healthily too – will re-stimulate that sense of marvel at what the body can do.

Contentment You learn to be thankful for your body's strength and health. Why does that matter? Because ultimately the fulfilled life is all about being content in yourself. And when we feel more positive, relaxed and accepting of all things, our lives feel in balance.

Pulling power The more attention you lavish on your body, the more at ease in it you feel. And the more at ease you are, the more attractive you are. A happy soul is far more beautiful and desirable than one who is self-critical and dissatisfied.

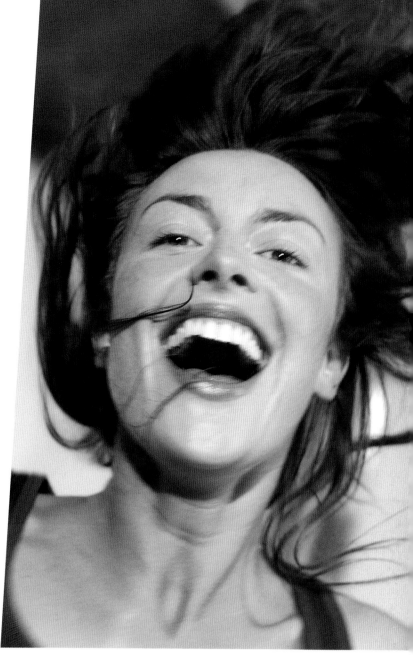

your bodycare kit

ALL THE ITEMS REQUIRED FOR THE MUST-DO
DAILY TRANSFORMERS ARE LISTED. ONCE
YOU'VE DECIDED WHICH BEAUTIFIERS AND
BOOSTERS MOST APPEAL TO YOU, PREPARE A
PERSONAL CHECKLIST OF OTHER ESSENTIALS
YOU'LL NEED, SO YOU HAVE EVERYTHING TO
HAND WHEN YOU MOST NEED IT.

Bath robe
Choose something easy you can slip into to
curl up and chill.

Music player
It must be battery operated because you can't
use a plug socket in the bathroom.

Candles
(and matches). It's the easiest way to dim
the lights and add atmosphere without
getting the electrician in. But next time you
redecorate, opt for dimmer switches in the
bathroom and bedroom.

Carrier oil
Choose almond oil, the perfect skin-
soothing oil to add to a bath if you have dry
or sensitive skin or to massage your hands
and feet.

Daily body moisturizer
Whether you opt for cream, lotion, gel or
serum, the lighter the product the less time
you generally need to allow for it to be
absorbed before dressing.

Energizing essential oils
Use lemon, orange, grapefruit, mandarin
and rosemary to sprinkle in your shower or
diffuse around your home as you wake up
and get ready for the day.

Flannel
You need this to wash your body briskly and
rev up your circulation.

Flip flops

You need them for padding around – you can do your pedicure in them – and they give you the feeling of an indulgent, pampering holiday.

Hair bands

Keep stray ends clean and dry.

Moisturizing shower wash

Available as cream, foam or gel, it's important because showers can be dehydrating to your skin.

Natural bristle body brush

Use to stimulate circulation all over your body first thing in the morning through dry body-brushing.

Relaxing essential oils

Add vetiver, geranium and lavender to your bath or diffuse around your home as you relax and unwind from the day.

Warm towels

Bath sheets are best: the bigger the towels, the more relaxed and comfortable you'll feel about your body.

For pedicure and manicure

You will need a pumice or foot file, a bowl, nail scissors , soft-cushion emery boards, cuticle cream, a rubber hoof stick, exfoliating cream or sea salt, toe dividers or cotton wool. Additional kit for manicure: cuticle remover, a nail brush, hand cream, nail-polish remover and a nail buffer.

transformers

Some prefer to shower and some prefer to bathe, but to maximize your bodycare regime and fully benefit from the products you use, you should do both. Use your morning shower ritual to scrub and clean your skin, your bedtime bathing ritual to soak, unwind and treat body and mind.

energizing morning ritual

QUICK, SKIN-TINGLING SHOWERS ARE THE BODYCARE EQUIVALENT TO A HANDSHAKE, WHILE BATHS ARE MORE OF A HUG. HOWEVER, MORNING WASH-DOWN SHOULD NEVER BE RUSHED. ADD A FEW EARLY-MORNING ENERGIZERS TO WAKE YOU UP AND REFRESH YOUR SKIN EACH DAY.

Before you even step in the shower, get into a new regime of **dry body-brushing**. It's an intense form of body exfoliation: as well as smoothing skin and boosting circulation, it's an invaluable part of your body's natural detoxification process, helping to stimulate the skin's lymphatic system and eliminate up to 30 per cent of the body's wastes.

A daily 5-minute workout will whisk away the dead skin cells which make skin look dry, dull and unhealthy. It will also help those lymph glands to flush out the toxins which are the main cause of cellulite, and quickly smooth rough, pimply uneven skin on the backs of arms, legs and buttocks.

Dry body-brushing should be done with a firm, natural bristle brush. Using upward, sweeping movements, you brush the entire body gently but firmly towards the heart. Start at the left foot, working up the leg to hip and abdomen. Repeat on the right side. Next brush from your right fingers, up your arm, across your shoulder and chest (avoid the nipples), and then across your back. Repeat on the left side. Finish by brushing down your neck towards your heart. Don't forget the detail as you go: brush between your fingers and toes, the inner thigh, and under the arms, where major lymph glands are located.

Don't miss Beauty therapists and models body brush within an inch of their lives. It's one of the most effective ways to get rid of cellulite. Make it part of your morning routine, much like brushing your teeth, for 14 days, and then every other day for the last week. Never brush skin that is broken or irritated. However, if you try body brushing and don't settle into the regime, do be sure to use a body exfoliator two or three times a week instead. Choose a grainy body exfoliator (the skin here isn't as sensitive as on your face, so you can use a coarser formulation), massage all over damp skin and rinse off.

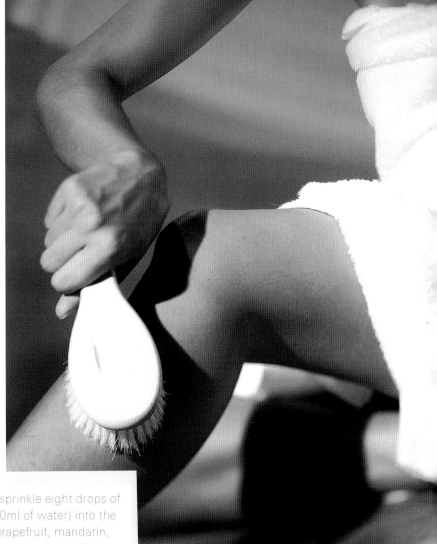

ALLOW 5 MINUTES FOR
YOUR LOTION TO DRY
BEFORE DRESSING.
CARRY OUT YOUR FACIAL
DAILY REGIME NOW.

Now **shower**. For a refreshing wake-up call, sprinkle eight drops of an invigorating, zesty essential oil (diluted in 50ml of water) into the shower tray before you turn on the spray. Try grapefruit, mandarin, orange or lemon – and rosemary is excellent if you really need to focus your mind (see page 220).

While you're luxuriating in the shower, try this exercise. for a count of 5, squeeze your buttocks together and pull in your abdomen as if you are trying to fit into a tight waistband. Relax and repeat five times. Do the exercise again, but this time press your knees and inner thighs together at the same time.

Wash with a **moisturizing** shower gel, cream or foam. Unlike bathing, where water is absorbed into your skin, showering removes surface oils under a torrent of water and this needs replacing. So it's vital to top up with moisture while you wash, and then have a body moisturizer ready to apply while your skin is damp, after towel-drying. Focus moisturizer (see page 125) on dry skin areas, such as the feet, shins, knees, elbows and chest

Need a boost? Once you've moisturized, you can focus a firming, slimming, anti-cellulite lotion on upper arms, abdomen, hips and thighs if you like. Skin-firming body lotions can't replace exercise and they don't eliminate cellulite. It's the focus of attention on problem areas and the combined effort of fitness, nutrition and massage rather than any cream alone that 'helps'. And they can give a psychological lift if you need encouragement as they temporarily tighten and smooth your skin.

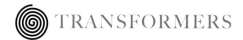
blissful bedtime ritual

Time to soak and bathe. The art of bathing is a much underrated mind/body therapy. With peace and solitude – family, please take note – where else can 20 minutes and a few aromatic additions give you the equivalent of two hours' rest and restoration?

When your body is very nearly immersed in warm water, nearly 90 per cent of its weight is displaced, so you instantly feel lighter and at ease. And you really will feel calmer too, as it lowers your blood pressure. A warm soak at the end of the day will also relax any muscle stiffness from unaccustomed exercise. Combine therapeutic body oils with these proven benefits and you create the perfect calming ritual to improve your quality of sleep.

Lower the lights and then **set the scene** with a scented candle or two. Turn the heating up and place a couple of bath towels over the radiator. Play some relaxing music. Run a warm bath. Wash your hands and feet before stepping in. If you plan to exfoliate or buff hard skin on your feet (using a grainy scrub or foot file), do so before bathing; afterwards the skin will be too soft and vulnerable. Now add a blissful oil blend to the water.

Normal to oily skin three drops each of vetiver, geranium and lavender pure essential oil (see page 220)
Dry or sensitive skin 10ml almond carrier oil and six drops of your favourite essential oil
Fragrance free six drops of soothing almond oil

Step in and **immerse yourself** in the warm water. Stay there for a full 20 minutes to benefit from the aromatherapy oils – no longer, or your skin will become dehydrated and crinkled.

Make the most of this 20 minutes of solitude with a **relaxation** technique. Place a rolled towel under your head and lie back. Close your eyes and inhale deeply through your nose to a count of 4 and then let out a long, low sigh. Breathing slowly and evenly (to the count of 4 each way), keep your eyes closed and focus on each part of your body in turn, working from your forehead down to your toes as you imagine 'letting go' any tension. Then allow your head to fill with a white light that represents all things warm, good and positive in your life. If any negative thoughts enter your mind, imagine the white light wrapping around them until there's only white light and peace left behind.

After bathing, dry yourself with a warm towel. Then **moisturize**, focusing on dry skin areas, such as the feet, shins, knees and elbows. Massage in creams, potions or oils to keep skin gleaming. Even if you've been neglectful, this can make a big difference in just seven of your 21 days.

Don't miss Bubble baths are drying on the skin – unless they're pH-balanced.

Fast track Use this time to have a face mask (see page 97) or place some soothing eye pads (see page 92) over your closed eyelids

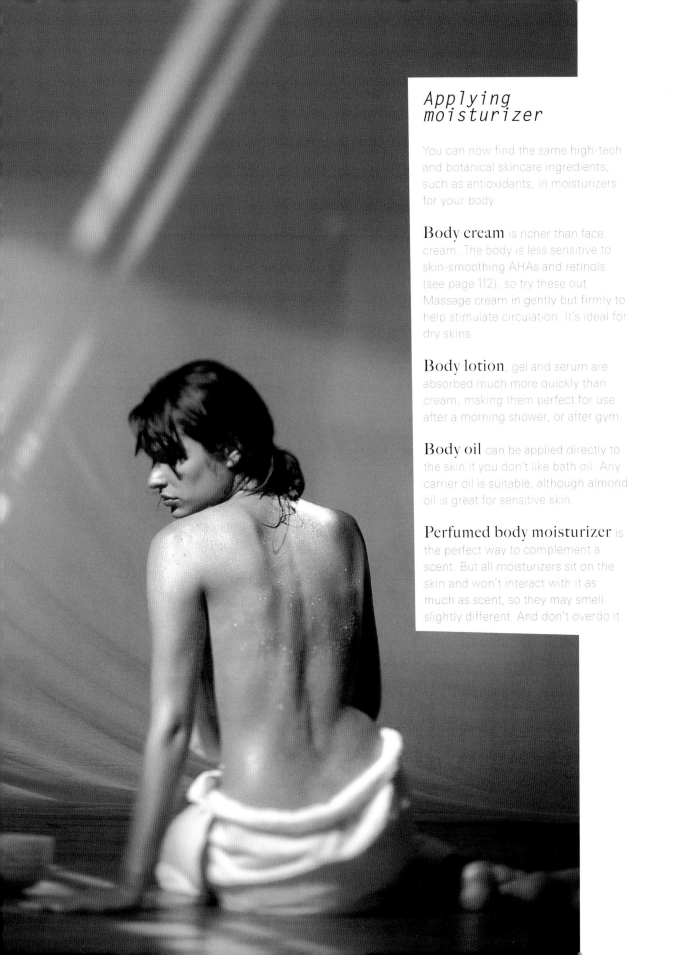

Applying moisturizer

You can now find the same high-tech and botanical skincare ingredients, such as antioxidants, in moisturizers for your body.

Body cream is richer than face cream. The body is less sensitive to skin-smoothing AHAs and retinols (see page 112), so try these out. Massage cream in gently but firmly to help stimulate circulation. It's ideal for dry skins.

Body lotion, gel and serum are absorbed much more quickly than cream, making them perfect for use after a morning shower, or after gym.

Body oil can be applied directly to the skin if you don't like bath oil. Any carrier oil is suitable, although almond oil is great for sensitive skin.

Perfumed body moisturizer is the perfect way to complement a scent. But all moisturizers sit on the skin and won't interact with it as much as scent, so they may smell slightly different. And don't overdo it.

beautifiers

With a little planning, you can add the benefits of a rejuvenating health-spa regime to your programme. Try to make time for one (or all) of these once-a-week body treats but allow four days between detoxers. Set aside half an hour for each one so you're not rushed.

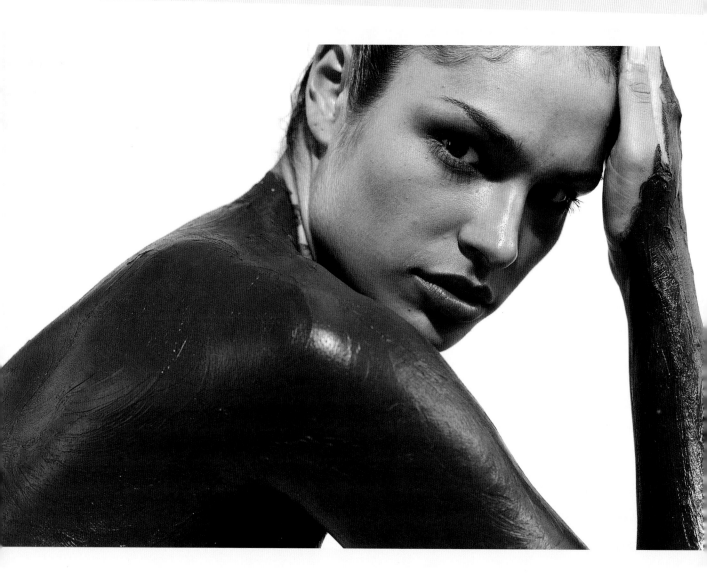

quick body-smoothing wrap

THIS ONE USES A BODY OIL YOU CAN BLEND FOR YOURSELF. IT'S 20 MINUTES OF PURE R&R AND A GREAT WAY TO HELP YOU WIND DOWN AFTER A PARTICULARLY STRESSFUL DAY.

Blend any combination of carrier oils, using olive, jojoba, hazelnut or almond, to make a 30ml base oil, and then add six drops each of anti-stress frankincense and vetiver pure essential oils. Keep in a dark glass bottle, using as much as you need.

1 Warm the oil between your palms and massage in all over your body at night, leaving it on your skin to be absorbed fully.

2 Wrap yourself up in a pre-warmed bathrobe and socks, and place a blanket over your lap. Sit back in a dimly lit room and practise some breathing exercises (see pages 211 and 224–5).

detoxifying mud wrap

THE HEALING PROPERTIES OF MUD HAVE BEEN USED FOR CENTURIES TO DEEP CLEANSE AND DETOXIFY. RICH IN MINERALS THAT CAN BE ABSORBED BY THE SKIN, MUD AND CLAY ARE EITHER TAKEN FROM THE SEA BED OR FROM THE EARTH. GREAT FOR WHEN YOUR BODY FEELS JADED OR STRESSED, A MUD WRAP ALSO MAKES A GOOD SLIMMING AID AS IT CAN HELP THE BODY ELIMINATE TOXINS FASTER.

Salon body mud-wraps involve being slathered in warm mud, and then wrapped up in layers of foil and blankets to keep in the heat and help draw out toxins. So be prepared: this is going to get very messy. Clay or mud for wraps can be bought at any good health-food shop. Some brands smell better than others too!

For this treatment, you need some extra kit: two old towels, one old sheet, one or two old blankets, and ideally a climber's silver insulating 'space' blanket. The more body heat you can trap, the more your skin will benefit from the warm mud.

1 Consider where you are going to lie down – on the floor or in an empty bath. I'd recommend the bath: the mess is rather more containable. Cushion with the towels and then, again to cut the mess factor, cover the whole area with the sheet.

2 Lay the space blanket (or an ordinary blanket) over the sheet, ready for you to lie on. Unfold the other blanket(s) and arrange on the edge of the bath within easy reach.

3 Follow the instructions to mix up a paste and, getting into the bath, apply to your skin immediately. Do it lying down, if you can.

4 Wrap the rest of the space blanket over you, and then flip the old blankets on top. Tuck your arm inside the blankets and relax. Allow the mud to dry (up to 20 minutes) before rinsing it off.

5 When you're ready to remove the mud, peel back the outer blankets carefully and drop onto the floor. Then unwrap the space blanket and, leaning forward in the bath, fold the sheet down over the space blanket to avoid dropping mud everywhere. Remove carefully to clean up later.

6 Stay in the bath and rinse the mud off, using a shower head, or run a warm bath and sponge it off.

7 Pat skin dry and follow with a body moisturizer. Your skin will feel soft and look so much brighter.

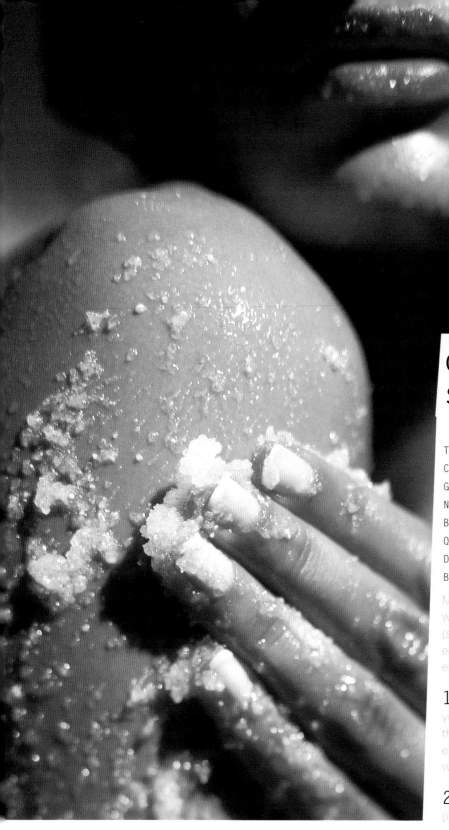

oil & salt scrub

THINK OF THIS AS A MUCH-NEEDED DEEP CLEANSE FOR YOUR BODY, HELPING TO GET RID OF ANY DRY OR BUMPY PATCHES. NEGLECTED SKIN (PARTICULARLY ON THE BOTTOM AND BACKS OF ARMS) RESPONDS QUICKLY TO A LITTLE EXTRA ATTENTION. DEAD SEA SALTS ARE AVAILABLE FROM BEAUTY SALONS AND BY MAIL ORDER.

Mix a handful of natural Dead Sea salts with pure almond or wheatgerm carrier oil (see page 220). You can add three drops each of lemon and rosemary pure essential oils for a stimulating effect.

1 Stand in the shower or bath and, with your skin slightly damp, concentrate on the upper back, shoulders, bottom, elbows and knees, massaging the scrub in with a gentle, circular movement.

2 Treat everywhere else on the body (including your hands and feet) with an even lighter action.

3 Shower off or run a warm bath and soak yourself to help detoxify the system.

deep-sea soak

BECAUSE THE OCEANS AND THE PLANTS THAT GROW IN THEM ARE SO RICH IN MINERALS, SEAWEED AND SEAWATER-BASED BODY TREATMENTS ARE EXCELLENT FOR DETOXIFYING THE BODY, STIMULATING THE METABOLISM AND REJUVENATING THE SOUL.

Seaweed (the generic name for marine algae) contains iodine (regulates the thyroid, protects skin against premature ageing and keeps hair strong), sodium and potassium (regulate cell fluid levels), iron (improves circulation) and copper (maintains skin and muscle fibre), and benefits your skin from the outside in.

1 Add your chosen marine algae/seaweed solution to your bathwater, and lie with your body submerged for about 20 minutes to allow the water to draw out impurities by osmosis. This lengthy soak also enables the many marine vitamins and minerals to be absorbed through your skin into your bloodstream.

2 When you emerge, pat your skin dry and follow with a body moisturizer or the body-smoothing wrap.

Variation Try a little hydrotherapy after your sea soak. This gently mimics ferocious jet spa treatments to boost circulation even more. Let the bath water run out and then spray your body vigorously with alternate 10-second bursts of very warm and cold water from the shower faucet ten times in all. Finish with a warm all-over body spray for a few minutes.

Cellulite is the name of that dimpled, orange-peel look on thighs, bottom and upper arms. It is said to affect around 80 per cent of women of every shape and size and level of fitness. The cause is not known, but one theory is that cellulite relates to the level of the female hormone oestrogen in the body, which is why it often hits hardest during puberty and pregnancy. Many experts believe that cellulite is a sign of long-term imbalances in the body, and is improved by cutting down on fat and sugar, drinking more water, and boosting the circulation and lymphatic system with regular exercise and massage.

Lymphatic system is the term given to your internal waste-removal system. Lymph circulates around the body, picking up waste and toxins and depositing them in the lymph glands. A build-up of waste due to poor circulation results in fatigue, water retention and even less effective circulation. Key lymph glands are found in your armpits and at the tops of your inner thighs.

Toxins disrupt the efficient functioning of our body systems. They are the product most notably of diet – sugar, food additives, alcohol, coffee, pesticides – along with stress, smoke and pollution. Toxic overload results from a consistent assault from all the above daily poisons, and your skin, eyes, hair and nails are often the first areas to be affected. Overload also results in fatigue, lethargy, temperamental behaviour – and more stress. It can eventually lead to problems of the bowel, bladder, liver and kidneys. Your Nutrition, Fitness and Relaxed Living chapters are invaluable if you suffer from toxic overload.

Detox (detoxification) literally means removing these toxic substances from your body. Many natural-health experts recommend detoxing for a couple of days each month, by drinking plenty of mineral water, avoiding wheat, dairy and sugary processed foods (that's days 3–7 of your Nutrition programme), and practising deep-breathing exercises to calm and relax the system. See the weekend spa programme set out on page 240 for a briefer detox plan. It's a useful follow-up routine.

boosters

Whenever you need a pick-me-up for your mind as much as your body, these sensational body boosters will make all the difference to the way you look within an hour, and instantly give the impression that you lavish your body with love and attention. Which, of course, now you do.

fake tan

MANY BELIEVE THAT TANNED SKIN LOOKS 4.5KG (10LB) LIGHTER AND FITTER THAN PALE SKIN. AND I, AS A FAIR-SKINNED REDHEAD, AGREE. BUT YOU MUST PROTECT THAT GORGEOUS SKIN FROM STRONG SUNLIGHT, SO PLAY SAFE AND FAKE IT.

All the lotions, creams and sprays are basically skin dyes, most of which contain the active ingredient dihydroxyacetone (DHA), which reacts with the proteins (amino acids) in the outer layers of your skin to produce a browning effect. Most results today are a great improvement on the orange colour still associated with fake tanning and offer a 'nearly natural' tan in hours. But do practise applying them before a hot date, especially if you are very pale, and never try out a new formula the day before you go on holiday.

If you've yet to try a fake-tanning product, here is a fool-proof method that suits even the whitest of skins. If you're still not convinced, buy a fake-tan product designed for the face and use that on your body. The overall colour will generally be much lighter.

1 Start by exfoliating your body all over (see page 128), paying particular attention to dry skin areas such as the knees and elbows that otherwise grab more of the dye and so end up looking darker.

2 Apply a moisturizing cream to these same dry areas. It will act as a slight barrier. Allow 5 to 10 minutes for it to absorb.

3 Apply fake-tan all over your body, massaging it in evenly. Wash your hands immediately. Leave to dry without touching anything for at least 15 minutes (it could be longer, depending on the brand you choose).

4 Allow 1 hour and then – regardless of how long the brand says to wait – take a shower. This ensures that any colour that hasn't been absorbed will wash away and you are less likely to end up with streaky, uneven patches.

Remember Many after-sun lotions now contain a tiny amount of DHA so they can give skin a subtle hint of colour too. Use them as a daily body moisturizer for an understated build-up of colour over several days.

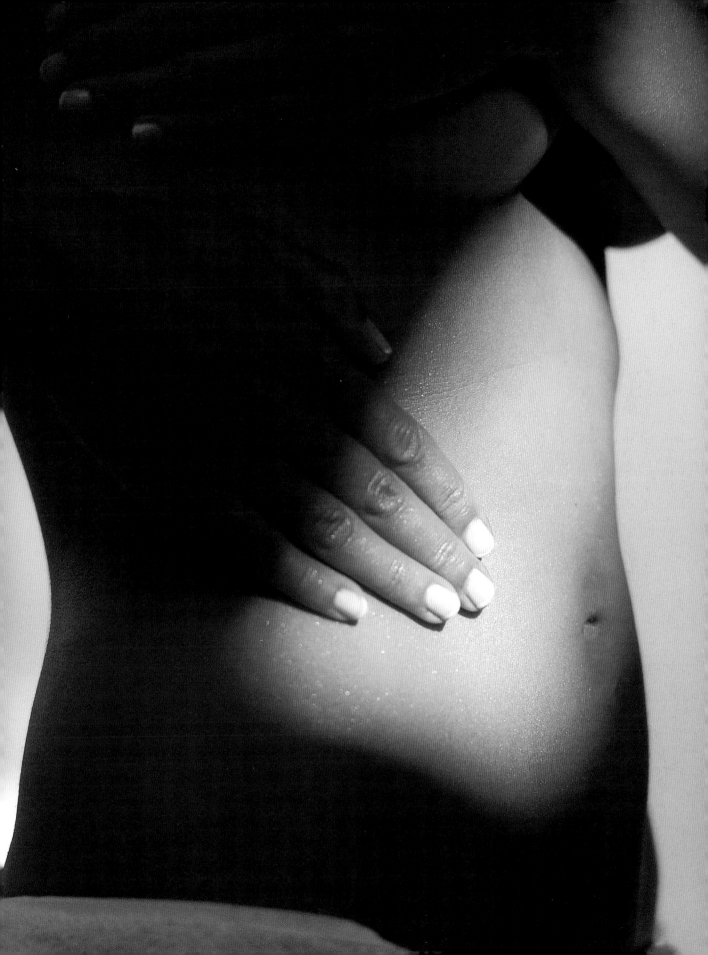

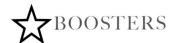

pamper pedicure

THERE'S SOMETHING VERY GROUNDING ABOUT WALKING AROUND BAREFOOT. CHIROPODISTS SAY WE SHOULD DO IT FOR AT LEAST 20 MINUTES A DAY FOR FOOT HEALTH, BUT I THINK IT'S A REAL FEEL-GOOD THING TOO. SOFT, SMOOTH FEET AND POLISHED TOES PADDING AROUND THE HOME ADD THAT LITTLE EXTRA SENSE OF 'WELL-GROOMED GORGEOUSNESS' WE ALL SEEK TO ACHIEVE.

We so rarely devote much time, care and attention to our feet. Yet just think what they do for us. When we walk a mile, we stride a thousand times and with each step each foot bears twice our body weight.

There are 72,000 nerve endings in each foot, wrapped around 28 bones – a quarter of all the bones in the adult body are in our feet – and those bones are held together by 38 muscles. That's what it takes to make our feet sensitive, yet strong and flexible enough to carry our weight in the arch and absorb the shock of impact on the sole with every step we take.

Now's the time, then, to take time – once a week will do – and treat your feet to a pampering pedicure. They are guaranteed to look and feel 100 per cent better than they did before. And they really can make a difference to the way you feel. Tired feet drag down the whole body so we shuffle around in a bad mood rather than skipping about light-footed.

Always paint your toenails

especially if you don't like your feet. It focuses on them, sure, but it always manages to make them look prettier. And even something as simple as choosing which colour to wear is a brief, yet feel-good moment.

What colour? No matter what colour you

go for, the skin next to the polish should appear to have a golden tinge. If your feet (or hands) look cold and grey, you've got the colour wrong. As a rough guide: redheads suit ambers, ochres, oranges, clear reds and peachy sheer; blondes suit pinks, pinky beiges and pale pink sheer; and brunettes suit plums, burgundy, royal blue, ruby, purple and white sheer. A French polish (see page 134) looks very pretty and stylish on toes.

1 Start by rubbing away hard dead skin from around the heels, balls of the feet and under the big toes with a pumice stone or foot file. Do this before soaking or showering otherwise you may remove too much skin and make the feet too sensitive.

2 Soak your feet in a bowl of warm water containing four drops of rosemary or lavender essential oil to deodorize and stimulate the circulation (as shown, a).

3 Trim the nails by cutting straight across to minimize risk of splitting or of in-growing toenails. Buff edges with the fine side of an emery board (as shown, b).

4 Use the rough side of an emery board to refine any dry skin around the toes.

5 Apply cuticle cream and massage into the base of each nail with your thumb pads. Wait a couple of minutes and then gently push back the cuticles, using a rubber hoof-stick or your thumb wrapped in a towel.

6 Massage exfoliating cream or damp sea salt all over your feet (as shown, c), using your fingertips in gentle, circular movements. Rinse and dry thoroughly.

7 Massage moisturizing cream into your feet, paying particular attention to the heels, and avoiding the areas between the toes, which should always be kept dry to prevent infection.

8 Inserting toe dividers (as shown, d) or cotton wool first, apply a clear, protein-rich base coat to help strengthen your nails and prevent splitting, flaking and staining from dark-coloured polish.

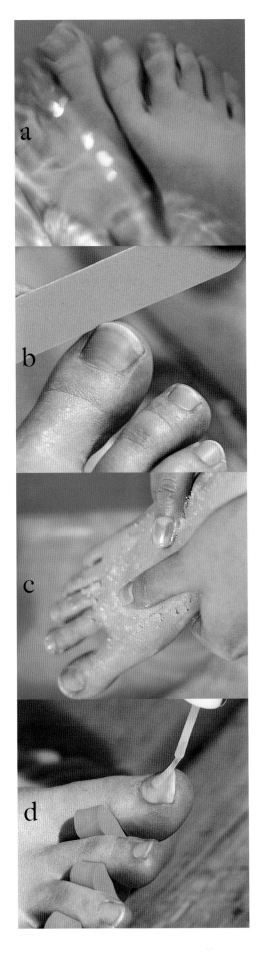

Anytime foot massage

JUST STROKING YOUR FEET HAS AN ENORMOUSLY UPLIFTING EFFECT ON YOUR WHOLE BODY. SO WHENEVER THEY'RE TIRED...

1   Place a couple of drops of almond oil between the palms of your hands to warm, smooth evenly over one of your feet and then make long, firm, thumb sweeps along the length of the sole from the arch to the toes.

2   Grasp the foot with one hand and rub the sole with the knuckles of your other hand.

3   Make small circles with your thumbs on the sole, massaging from the ball of the foot down to the heel.

4   Rub away any last tension on the foot with fingertip strokes.

5   Hold the toes with one hand and the heel with the other and wring the foot by twisting your hands in opposite directions.

6   Repeat on the other foot.

Relaxing treat Soak your feet in a bowl of warm water with a couple of drops each of geranium and lavender pure essential oils to soothe aching arches after a long day.

Don't miss If your feet are really dry, the best treatment is to smother them in petroleum jelly and wear old socks all night. Not recommended on hot summer nights, but it's guaranteed to improve the roughest of feet by morning.

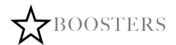

your 10-minute manicure

YOUR HANDS SAY SO MUCH ABOUT YOU. BUFFED AND POLISHED, THEY REFLECT GOOD GROOMING. UNPROTECTED AND UNKEMPT, THEY SUGGEST THAT YOU JUST DON'T CARE. AND EVEN IF YOUR HANDS AREN'T THE GREATEST SHAPE, YOU CAN ALWAYS IMPROVE ON THE LOOK OF YOUR NAILS. IT TAKES LESS TIME THAN YOU'D THINK AND IT'S THERAPEUTIC TOO – SPENDING LOVING TIME CARING FOR YOURSELF THROUGH YOUR HANDS.

1 Use scissors to cut your nails into a straight shape – never clippers, which shatter the nail and cause the end to split

2 File with a gentle, soft-cushion emery board (not a metal file)

3 Rub cuticle cream in the nail area and then place your hands in a bowl of warm water and soak for 2 minutes

4 Dry your hands and apply cuticle remover if required (leave on for no longer than 2 minutes)

5 Gently push back and neaten the cuticles with a hoof stick. Neat cuticles (the bits around the nail that get dry and you might feel inclined to chew or tear) are the making of any manicure

6 Soak your hands again (for 2 minutes) and then scrub your nails gently with a brush to remove any last traces of dirt or cuticle cream. Dry your hands and massage in hand cream. Leave for 3 minutes, and then rub a little nail polish remover over your nails to remove any hand cream residue.

7 Lightly buff the surface of your nails with the grainy side of a nail buffer and then rub smooth, using the smooth side. Now your nails are smooth and shiny – ready to leave bare and beautiful or to paint.

Don't miss Why special hand cream? It's usually less greasy than other creams so it absorbs quickly. If you make hand cream part of your Bodycare regime every time you wash your hands, you'll notice a difference within 14 days. And keep a tube in your bag, car, office, and by your bed too.

French polish A French manicure gives the perfect healthy, groomed but natural look to nails (hands or feet). The nail tips are painted white (keep a steady hand and remove any mistakes with a cotton bud dipped in nail varnish remover), and then the entire nail is coated in a pale pink.

Anytime hand relaxer

HANDS GET STRESSED OUT TOO. USE THIS AS A TIME TO MASSAGE IN PLENTY OF HAND CREAM.

1 Form your hands into clenched fists, hold for a few seconds and release, straightening the fingers out as you do so. Repeat 10 times. Feels good, doesn't it?

2 Clasp your hands with fingers tightly interlocked. Press both fingers and palms together as firmly as you can for a count of 5. Release and shake your fingers vigorously. Repeat ten times.

3 Place your palms together as if in prayer, but facing outward away from your body. Then lift your palms so that only the fingers and thumbs remain in contact with each other. Press for a count of 3 and release. Repeat ten times.

4 Finish by gentle pulling along each finger, using the other hand in a quick, 'flick' action. There's no need to crack joints – the idea is to release tension and relax your hands.

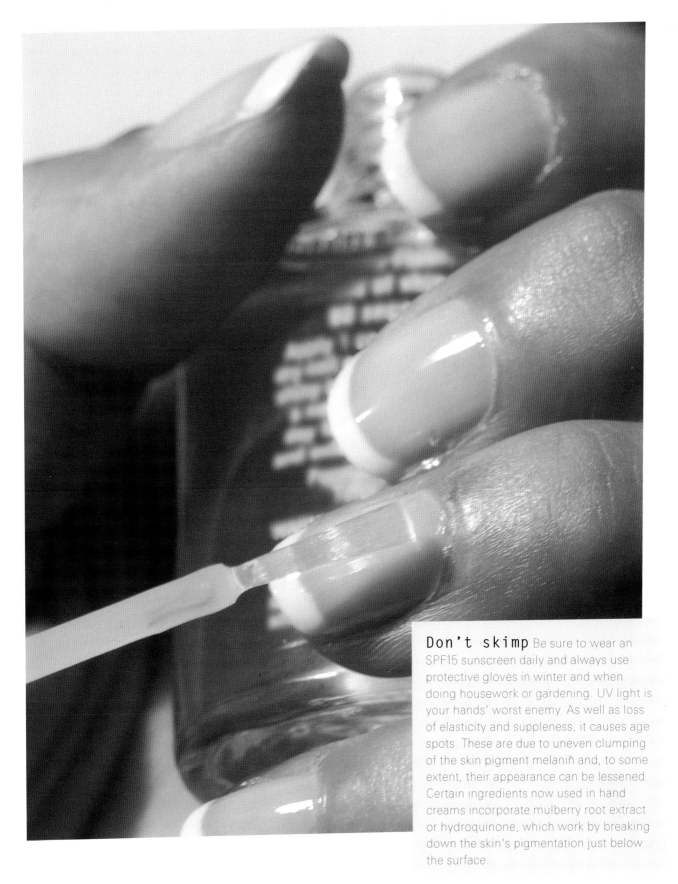

Don't skimp Be sure to wear an SPF15 sunscreen daily and always use protective gloves in winter and when doing housework or gardening. UV light is your hands' worst enemy. As well as loss of elasticity and suppleness, it causes age spots. These are due to uneven clumping of the skin pigment melanin and, to some extent, their appearance can be lessened. Certain ingredients now used in hand creams incorporate mulberry root extract or hydroquinone, which work by breaking down the skin's pigmentation just below the surface.

Prefer a morning bath? Add a couple of handfuls of coarse sea salt to the water. It will lightly scrub your skin and leave you feeling wonderfully restored.

No time to redo your polish? Carefully dab in polish to cover the smear or chip, using several thin layers in the same colour, and then apply two coats over the entire nail.

Sunburned or itchy skin? Have a lukewarm bath and add three drops of camomile and five drops of lavender pure essential oils to soothe and heal.

Puffy ankles? Give them a good soak – immerse your feet up to the ankles, in hot and then cold water to reduce swelling fast.

Uneven toenails? A French polish on your feet (see page 134) can magically neaten up uneven nail lengths to give the illusion of naturally perfect feet.

Goose flesh? Use a circulation booster to kick-start your system into action each day. Dry body-brushing is very good, or use a body exfoliator, such as a loofah, in the bath or shower, or a body scrub.

fast track

Feeling tired? Yawn deeply and loudly. It's your body's way of getting more oxygen to the brain and it increases mental clarity.

Perfect nails If left to dry properly (at least half an hour to an hour), polish will always last longer.

Prone to bumps and bruises? Try the homeopathic remedy, arnica, when you knock yourself and you'll suffer less bruising. Apply as a topical cream or take tablets.

Try a mud bath Bought from all good health shops and beauty departments, these baths look less than inviting, but the effect is extremely uplifting. Stay in the water for the full 20 minutes, and sip a cup of hot water or cleansing fennel tea to boost the detoxifying effects. Shower off quickly afterwards, cosy up, rest and relax.

Aching muscles afer a workout? Soak your body in a warm bath to which you've added a blend of pure essential oils: two drops of black pepper*, three drops of frankincense and one drop of rose otto. *Avoid if you have high blood pressure.

Treat yourself to a mini massage Do it any time you're applying cream, lotion or oil: it gets your circulation going and improves the lymphatic system. Start at your head and face, and work down your neck, shoulders, arms, torso, hips and legs to the bottom of your feet.

keeping it going

Seek balance

Stay grounded by still walking barefoot around your home each morning. When you're stressed, the adrenal glands go into hyperdrive. Practise simple deep-breathing techniques, meditation or yoga – all help to induce a state of calm (see chapter 7).

Choose a better path

Don't forget that the look of your body has more to do with your lifestyle choices than your age. This means that everything you eat and drink, how much sleep and exercise you get, how much stress you have in your life, together with what you put on your skin, will determine its appearance. So use your now you plan as a constant support.

● Moisturize your body inside and out. Getting enough moisture is vital for plump, glowing, healthy-looking skin. Layer moisturizer on your skin after bathing and showering until it becomes routine. Get into the habit of drinking more water – have an occasional glass of hot water with a slice of lemon instead of your mid-morning or mid-afternoon coffee – it's refreshing, thirst-quenching and skin-toning.

● At least once a week – without fail! – indulge in a skin-boosting treatment, such as a foot massage, an oil & salt scrub or a deep-sea soak. Paying attention to yourself in this way means you're far less likely to ignore your skin's needs, and getting into the habit of lavishing care on your body continues to build your confidence and self-esteem.

● Exercise more (see page 76). Many more people are becoming overweight at a much younger age. Long-term effects of obesity include diabetes, heart disease, and muscle, joint and back problems.

● Help your body to detox itself. Remember: poor circulation leads to a build-up of waste in the lymph glands, resulting in fatigue, water retention and poor skin tone. Any body massage is therapeutic. Find the key lymph glands at the tops of your inner thighs and in your armpits and spend a few minutes each day massaging them when you're rubbing in moisturizer.

● Always get the day off to a good start by not rushing your morning rituals. It's so much better to wake just half an hour earlier. Keep up those early-morning energizers (such as zesty essential oils in the shower basin), the early-morning stretches (page 58) and/or your wake-up moments (page 208) and you'll rise more refreshed with each day.

● Remind yourself that the sun is ageing and make an effort to protect your hands and chest from now on – these are the areas where age spots first appear. Wear a wide-brimmed hat and a sunblock, and top up the fake tan regularly.

● If your hands tend to be dry, never again do the washing up or cleaning without rubber gloves.

● Stay aware of your body: make sure you recognize its signals and respond.

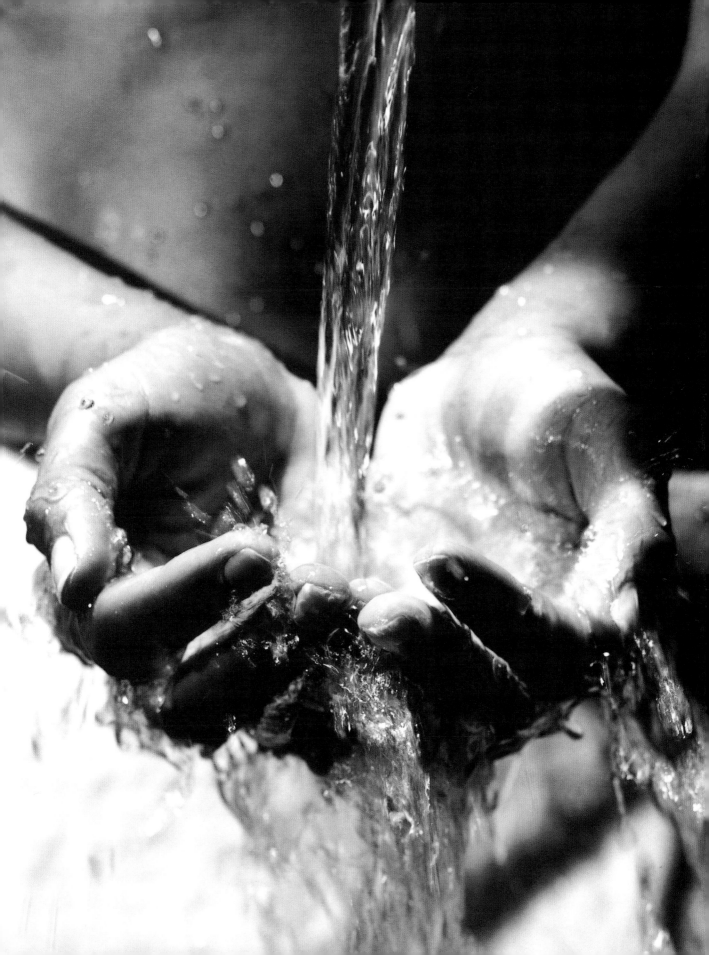

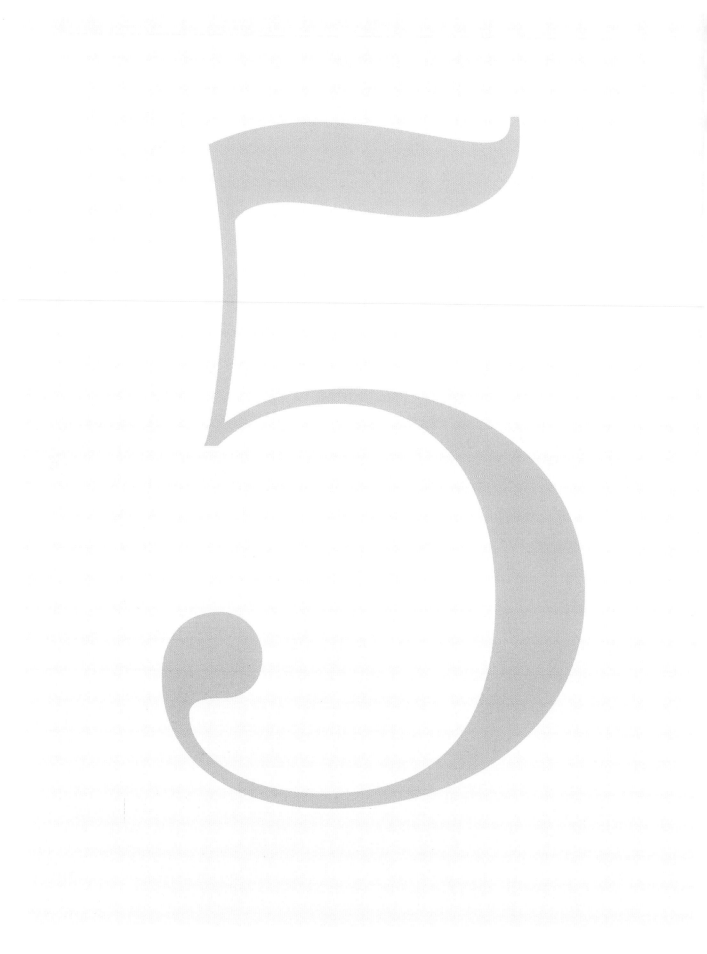

21 DAYS

TO

GREAT

MAKE-UP

It's about making the very best of what you've got. The pure pleasure of applying make-up will have you feeling just as good as you look.

Your
make-up
programme

Make-up can't change your life, but it can light up your face and add a much-needed bloom and radiance to your skin. Better still, with this part of the plan you don't even have to wait 21 days to see an improvement. But totally instant it's not. Applied badly, make-up can sink into creases, accentuate each fine line and make you wish you hadn't bothered. So practise a little.

BEING COMFORTABLE WITH A LOOK IS ONE THING: STICKING WITH IT FOR A DECADE IS ANOTHER.

Time for change? Take a much closer look at yourself. Do you look the way you did ten years ago? One way a woman can really age herself is with her make-up. Aim to change lifelong make-up rituals over the next 21 days. Ask yourself how you want to look, who do you aspire to look like. Be realistic about what you can achieve. My advice? Stick to classic. Whatever your skin colour or its texture, the make-up that sits quietly on your skin – so you look better but no one around you knows quite why – is timeless, go-anywhere make-up.

Remember Accept your uniqueness. Play always to your positives. And less is very much more.

Haven't worn make-up for years? Then stay with something simple, such as the fast-track regime. Get into the habit of applying it every morning on a freshly cleansed and moisturized face – without fail – and you'll soon get used to the feeling of being groomed. It takes less time than you think to bring out the best in your face.

Time to experiment But don't feel under pressure to use every single item and technique described here. The purpose of this programme is to teach you a few tricks that you can include in your day – whether you already wear make-up or not. Whatever your style, decide to try something new, even if it's just a different shade of lipstick. Learn how to wear eyeliner if you've resisted it until now. What about curling your lashes as a matter of course? Arch and sculpt your brows so they look more elegant. You'll be amazed the difference cosmetics can make.

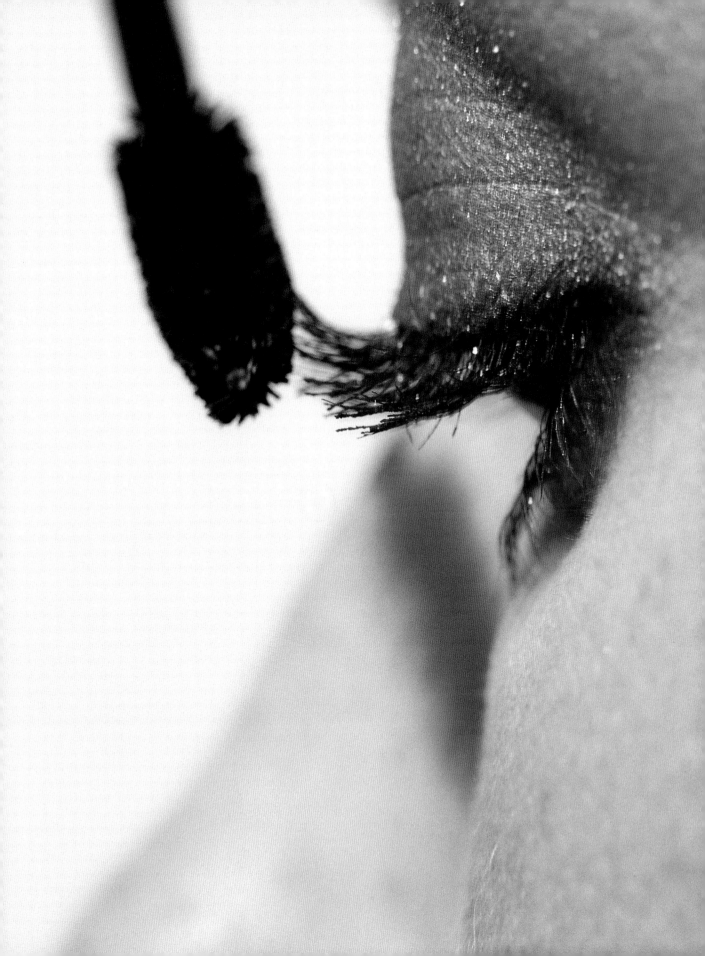

What you do in these 21 days

if you're 20-35...

Your skin is still young, firm and smooth enough to allow you to experiment with fashion make-up trends. Now is the time to practise application techniques. Remember that classic make-up never goes out of fashion. And don't neglect your Nutrition and Skincare programmes, majoring on anything – weekly masks, steams and scrubs – that will help your skin maintain its youthful radiance.

● Find a good base that matches your skin tone. Tune into your skin now and you'll understand it better over time.
● You like your make-up to look modern and fresh. Gloss and shine say youth so apply it well.
● Add colour or camouflaging concealer to counteract lack of sleep. Late nights take their toll on radiance.

...35-50

You still like your make-up to look fresh and modern, but no longer need to wear make-up just to be 'in'. You're looking rather to enhance your features, which are starting to losing their youthful bloom. Make-up may often mask imperfections, but powder will exaggerate dryness, and cream settles in fine lines. Remember to boost nourishing and softening skincare routines.

● Master the fast track make-up regime. You can't get away with no make-up any more, but these key grooming essentials are the basics you need if time is short.
● Wear foundation. You probably need a bit of base to even out your skin tone, and it acts as an added daily sunscreen.
● Make blusher your number one ally now – it replaces the colour that's beginning to fade from your cheeks.
● Boost your nourishing and softening skincare routines.

...50 and over

Subtlety is the key. Your skin has more wrinkles and the overall texture will have slackened. Now is the time to be even more confident in the make-up base you use. But hormonal changes mean that your skin may well feel much drier so a super-moisturizer under make-up and regular pampering with moisturizing facials are vital.

● Rethink your make-up. Be cautious with powder. It has a tendency to settle into wrinkles and exaggerate them.
● Establish a new colour code. Your natural colouring is probably undergoing a change – paler skin or lighter coloured, greying hair means it is time to establish a whole new look. Brows and lashes fade along with your hair colour, so where once you wore black mascara, now wear a natural-looking brown. And where you once wore a youthful pink blusher, now make it a softer, tawny pink.
● Stick to semi-sheer, semi-matt for foundation, powders and lipsticks. Matt textures flatten and deaden mature skins, and very shiny textures highlight any skin that isn't smooth.

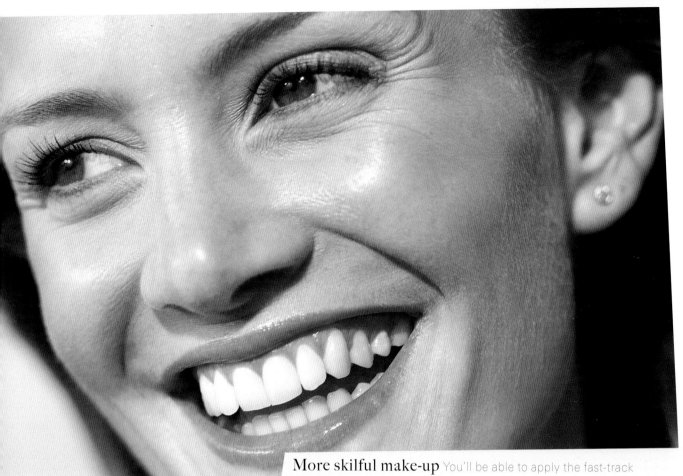

What you'll achieve

More skilful make-up You'll be able to apply the fast-track make-up confidently and know how to spend longer on your face when you need to present a more glamorous image. You'll appreciate the way make-up can change your look in minutes and feel inclined to go out more often too. This has to enhance your life – and your relationships with others.

Understanding Learning how to apply make-up more skilfully will help you get to know your skin better. Because through the process of finding a make-up regime that suits your skin, you recognize how it changes from morning to night, summer to winter.

Higher self-esteem You've indulged yourself, focusing on your self-image. The more attention you lavish on you, the more self-assured, the more sexy, you will feel. By paying attention to make-up application techniques, using special products to enhance or conceal, your confidence has truly begun to soar. (And if you've been diligent with your Skincare programme, you'll soon be wearing less concealer too, because the better your skin looks, the less you need to cover it up.)

Sure, make-up is only cosmetic – and superficial. But it's also the quickest way to give yourself an emotional and physical lift when you're feeling tired or low. Grooming says 'I care' to you and to those around you. And when you know you look more groomed, you feel more confident. Make-up has power.

your make-up kit

Indispensable

ALL THE ITEMS REQUIRED FOR THE MUST-DO
DAILY TRANSFORMERS ARE LISTED. ONCE
YOU'VE DECIDED WHICH BEAUTIFIERS AND
BOOSTERS MOST APPEAL TO YOU, PREPARE A
PERSONAL CHECKLIST OF OTHER ESSENTIALS
YOU'LL NEED, SO YOU HAVE EVERYTHING TO
HAND WHEN YOU MOST NEED IT.

Blusher
Go for a neutral pinky beige to imitate the
effects of a bracing walk in the fresh air.
Stick to creams on bare skin, and powder
on powdered skin.

Brow pencil
It should be mid brown in colour, and waxy so
it doesn't smudge, but still blends.

Clear lipgloss
(lip balm if you prefer). This gives a youthful
look and isn't often drying. It can be used to
add fullness to thin lips and mixed with your
favourite lip colour to create a glossier, more
sheer texture.

Concealers
The one you use on your face needs to be
yellow-toned to blend in best with your skin
tone. Use a special, light-reflecting under-eye
concealer to minimize dark shadows – the one
you use for the rest of your face may contain
an anti-bacterial ingredient that you shouldn't
place near your eyes.

Concealer brush
This tiny, finely pointed, short-bristled brush is
easy to control so you cover only what you
need to.

Dark brown mascara
It's more forgiving than black. Choose a glossy,
sheer formula that enhances lashes without
making them look too intense.

Fingertips
Provided they're clean, your fingertips are one
of the best make-up tools as they perfectly
contour your features and can gently pat and
press foundation, shadow and blusher into
place.

Lip colour
It comes in many different textures as
well as colours, and changes your look
in seconds.

Loose powder

It must be superfine for the sheerest, matt effect along the T-zone. Keep cheeks powder free for a fresher look.

Metal eyelash comb

Use it to separate each lash and remove clumps of mascara – 100 per cent better than any plastic comb.

Mid brown eyeshadow

Use a neutral shade to contour the eyes around the socket, and it doubles as brow powder for almost every hair colour.

Neutral eyeshadow

This matt eyeshadow, anything from pale ivory or beige to a mid brown for darker skin, should closely match your skin colour.

White eyeshadow

Choose one with a slight shimmer to highlight and illuminate the eyes, and to help shape and enhance darker areas. Use on the browbone or centre of the lid to make eyes sparkle.

Makes a big difference

Blusher brush Softly tapered sides can add subtle layers of colour to the cheeks.

Eyebrow brush Short, firm, angled bristles allow for clean, even application.

Eyeliner Use to emphasize eyes and to give the impression of fuller lashes.

Eyeliner brush A finely tipped brush, it is used to paint on liquid or block/cake liner.

Eyeshadow brush This short brush places colour exactly where you want it.

Foundation This will smooth and even out every type of skin.

Lipbrush Used to apply lipstick from the tube, you get a better shape and use less.

Lipliner Add shape to your mouth without too obvious a line round your lips.

Metal tweezers Angled and pointed, they will rarely miss a single hair.

Powder brush Sweep over the face to lighten the amount of powder used.

Velour powder puff It smoothes and softens the appearance of powder on skin.

transformers

The 'right' make-up for you will always depend on your lifestyle. It should be whatever you need it to be, whenever the time of day. But the aim is always the same: to enhance what you see in the mirror just enough and so subtly that only you know it's make-up.

fast-track make-up

DOES A SLICK OF LIPSTICK USUALLY SEE YOU FINE OUT OF THE HOUSE? WELL, TRY THIS SIMPLE UPGRADE: POWDER TO STOP SHINE OVER THE T-ZONE, EYELINER AND MASCARA IF YOUR EYES NEED DEFINITION, LIPGLOSS AND A FLUSH OF BLUSHER. JUST FIVE MINUTES IS ALL IT TAKES.

Loose powder makes skin look soft and velvety, minimizes pores and absorbs excess shine. And that's great for the T zone if you have oily or combination skin. If your skin is dry, you need a light application otherwise it will emphasize lines. So, whatever your skin type, get a big brush and swirl it over your face for 2 seconds. Be selective about where you powder: the forehead, nose and/or chin. Always leave cheeks powder free. And never rub powder onto the skin – it will settle too heavily in the pores and the creases.

Don't miss Check if powder particles have settled in your eyebrows or lashes. If they have, brush through immediately.

Must have **lipstick**. Even those who rarely use foundation or blusher wear it. It can be an intense colour that lasts for hours, or a shorter-lived, easy-going gloss. For your fast-track make-up, go for a creamy tinted gloss in pinky or berry nude shades. It's simple to touch up throughout the day – even without a mirror – so you'll never be left with an unattractive lipline.

Don't skimp How well lipstick goes on and stays on has a lot to do with the way you prime your lips. Dry lips soak up emollients, while leaving behind an uneven stain, whereas an overly moist mouth means that even the longest-lasting formula will slide off in real time. Keep using that lip balm.

Need definition? After the powder...

Keep **eyeshadow** simple. A clean sweep of one matt colour that closely matches your skin tone is all you need for a basic, groomed daytime look. Optional: add a hit of shimmer on the browbone or centre of the eyelid to look as if you've 'done more'

Not everyone needs **eyeliner** and if you have to devote a good 5 minutes to the job – you haven't got the time. So if you can get away with just mascara, do it. However, as lashes become sparse and eyes become deeper with age, eyeliner is indispensable (see page 154 for application tips).

One flick of the wand and **mascara** thickens and emphasizes your lashes – it's the most essential item of make-up for almost every woman. A good mascara is one that stays looking glossy once it's dried. Dull lashes just don't look healthy. For the best result, apply two fine coats to freshly curled lashes rather than one quick, thick coat. Your lashes are less likely to cake and stick together. Wipe the wand first with a tissue, and then brush the upper lashes downward from the top, and upward from the bottom. Avoid mascara on lower lashes – it's more inclined to smudge. Finish by brushing through with a metal eyelash comb. Replace mascara every six weeks, dry, clumpy mascara is ageing.

Don't skimp If you have pale lashes, use liquid eyeliner in a matching shade to fill in the lash base. This trick makes sparse lashes look thicker too.

AFTER YOUR DAILY SKIN REGIME, EAT YOUR BREAKFAST AND ALLOW YOUR SKINCARE TO BE FULLY ABSORBED. THEN APPLY YOUR MAKE-UP. IT'LL STAY IN PLACE BETTER.

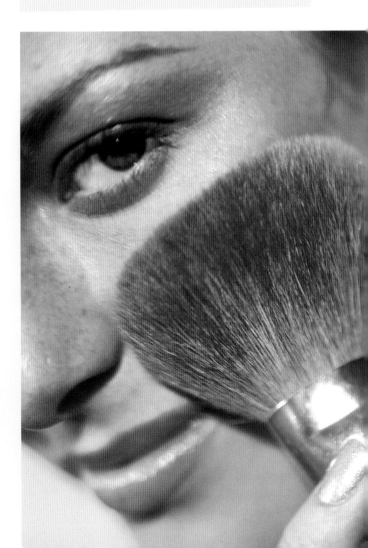

Blusher is the other essential item. It's the best remedy for the signs of stress and fatigue, and can give your skin a quick boost mid-afternoon. Lightly dusted over your cheekbones, chin and eyelids, a pinky fawn blush adds youth, warmth and vitality in just one step.

Blusher looks best when you apply it to the apple of your cheek. Powder blushers are easy to apply with a big fluffy brush and make retouching easy – dust in a circular motion. Creams are best on oilier skins or skin that's free from powder. Avoid gel blushers, these dry so quickly that they stain skin before you can blend them.

Remember It's easier to build up colour than take it away. If you overdo blusher, use a damp cosmetic sponge to blend in a little foundation, and then dab on a little powder to blend.

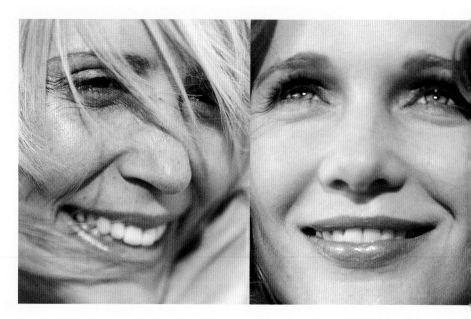

your ideal colours

I'm not into making rules for anyone, but there's little doubt that certain make-up shades suit certain colourings. If in doubt, you can't go wrong with basic, neutral, skin-tone shades. Use this as a rough guide to which classic colours really suit you best.

Blondes

Hair colour ranges from platinum blonde (and grey), through natural honey-golden blonde and olive-skin with highlights to ash blonde. Blonde hair requires a light touch with make-up and softer colours than you might imagine.

Base Foundation and/or powder should be lightweight and yellow-toned to match your skin tone and skin type exactly.

Cheeks should be soft (whether you're a natural blonde or not). Cool pinks, plum and rosy-beige blusher will give a natural flush. Warm pinks, peach and coral look good with a tan.

Eyes that are pale come to life with dark shadows, such as charcoal, deep lavender, brown or navy. Ivory, champagne and gold are pretty with warmer-toned skin.

Lips can get away with both pale and deep shades. Peach with a just hint of brown and warm browny reds are great for dark blondes, while berry, peachy brown, cappuccino brown and soft bubblegum are good for fair blondes.

Redheads

Naturally fair skinned and prone to freckles, redheads need yellow-toned base colours to counteract a natural pinkiness. Sheer make-up in warm subtle shades works best.

Base Foundation and/or powder should be light in texture to keep freckles looking fresh rather than covered up. A tinted moisturizer will even out skin tone.

Cheeks suit tawny, apricot and peachy brown shades.

Eyes that are pale need gold, terracotta and coppery brown. Brown eyes suit taupe, coffee and bronze better.

Lips can range through terracotta, peachy browns and berry tones. Sheer lips are great for day, berry tones for evening.

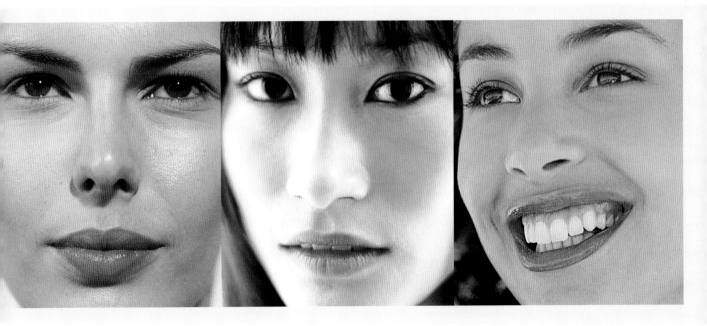

Brunette

Colouring can vary considerably. Be guided by your hair and skin colours, which are either warm or cool. Do you tend to suit gold or platinum and silver best? It's often a good indication.

Base Yellow-toned foundation and/or powder suits most types.

Cheeks Cool pinks and pale plums will define and complement a cool skin tone. Terracotta and tawny blusher are a better choice for a warmer skin tone.

Eyes can go dramatic. Practise the smoky-eye technique (see page 158) with shades of chocolate brown and black eyeliner and mascara. If your skin is pale, you can wear cool colours – lilac, lavender, aquas, taupe and cool browns. Olive skin and dark eyes suit taupe, deep brown, warm olive and charcoal.

Lips can range from pinky brown, heather and plum to a true red for cool brunettes, while olive-skinned brunettes suit toffee, cinnamon and browny reds.

Oriental

The skin of those with oriental colouring is often smooth and apparently poreless, pale yet warm in tone, and ages well.

Base Foundation and/or powder should be very fine and sheer, and match your yellow-based skin tone. Choose translucent or peach powder to add luminosity.

Cheeks need pink or plum blusher. Use just under the apple of the cheek to shape a round face.

Eyes that are deep and dark are often best defined by classic neutral shades, such as ivory, taupe, coffee and beige. Black eyeliner is a must, and avoid coloured mascara.

Lips can go light and sheer, looking good in pinks, pinky brown and plum shades.

Black

So-callled black skin varies greatly from light brown to very dark brown.

Base Finding a good base is the hardest task of all. Deep yellow tones suit the majority of black skins – with a hint of mahogany if your skin is very dark. Avoid powders which contain too much white – these will simply look grey. Choose a cosmetics brand that caters well for dark skin to find your perfect match. And remember: if it's a match, it should disappear into your skin.

Cheeks Use warm peach or cinnamon blusher for subtle definition. A little highlighter on the tops of the cheeks and browbones is flattering for evening.

Eyes look good in a wide range of colours. If you have warm golden or reddish tones in your hair, brown eyes will look more striking with golden browns, copper and warm beige. Dark brown eyes, with black skin and black hair, can wear purples and reds, as well as shimmery beige and charcoal. The latter is your ideal choice for eyeliner.

Lips suit sheer coffee browns, berry tones and nude shades of beige and pink gloss. Shimmery lip balm conditions and looks stunning on black skin.

make-up for day

When you need to make more of an impression, when you need a regime that will keep you looking good all day long – aim to look classically groomed. Wear barely-there, neutral shades, avoid obvious colour and play up your best features.

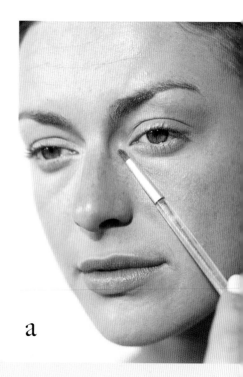

a

1   Skin always looks its best when you cover up only what you need to, leaving the rest of your skin clear. Dip a very fine, pointed brush in a perfectly matched foundation or concealer, and paint out all imperfections. After applying foundation, wipe any excess from your cheeks to leave as much natural colour as possible for a more youthful look.

2   Women of a certain age need eye concealer. Choose one that lightens dark areas around the eyes rather than covering them with a heavy layer. Look straight ahead into a mirror, lower your chin, and apply only to the dark areas (as shown, a).

3   If you need powder, use it in the T-zone: the centre of the forehead, nose and chin.

4   Ensure eyes are primed with a layer of face powder to absorb surface oils and to help eyeshadow stay put. Apply a neutral powder eyeshadow to match your natural skin tone) over the entire eyelid, blending up to the browbone (as shown, b). Take another neutral shadow, one shade darker, and apply along the socket of the eye and blend well so the two shades merge.

5   Brush the darker shade through your brows. Groom brows into place with a slick of brow gel if you have it.

6   For a discreet daytime eyeliner, take a pencil liner and draw along the underside of the lower lashes. Finish with mascara on the upper lashes (as shown, c, and see also page 149).

7   For the perfectly defined mouth, prime your lips with lip balm (as shown, d). If needed, shape (see page 160), using a lipliner that matches the colour of your lips, and soften the edges with a clean cotton bud. Apply colour, using a lipbrush. Then blot with a tissue and add another layer of colour.

8   Creamy blushers are great for summer and on cheeks free from make-up, but powder gives a more lasting finish. Swirl a blusher brush over the apple of your cheeks and blend away into the hairline beside them.

In summer

● Tinted moisturizers, creams and lipgloss come into their own and you can wear less. Fake tan affects the colour balance of your make-up.
● Swap blusher for bronzing powder for a sun-kissed look. Pick a shade that brightens your skin to the shade you'd turn naturally. Apply it on top of powder so it won't cake or smear. Think where the sun hits your face – the bridge of the nose, tops of cheeks, and browbones – and use it only there.
● Creamy blusher looks great on summer skin that's free from powder. Start on the apple of your cheeks and slowly work outwards, diffusing it at the edges so it blends away.
● Waterproof mascara is essential in summer but it contains volatile oils that evaporate on application to leave a hard, shiny coating on your lashes. (This makes it tricky to remove – you'll need an oily make-up remover.)
● A tube of powder-based T-zone controlling gel or cream can be applied over your make-up base along the T-zone, so touch-ups are easy.

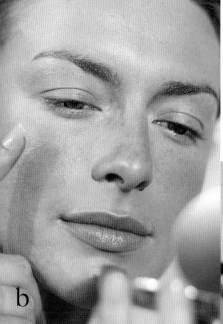

b

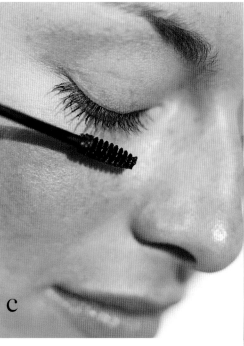

c

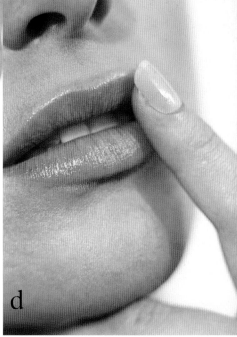

d

In winter

● Blusher looks unnatural if it doesn't tone with your natural skin shade, especially in winter when skin usually pales. Try to match your blusher as closely as possible with the colour of your cheeks.
● Remember the skincare and nourish your lips with a moisturizing balm. Accentuate your eyes instead.
● If you suffer from high colour but want to apply blusher, try calming with a hint of concealer, and then choose a tawny peach blusher rather than a pink shade. Remember: you're better off living with high colour than trying to hide it completely or your skin will just end up looking grey.
● Colours become deeper and richer, textures more matt and defined, to go with heavier, darker fabrics and the weather. But wear what suits you.

make-up for night

When you need more drama for something special, think quality NOT quantity. Aim to look sophisticated in an understated way. Wear neutral tones similar to your daytime make-up – only a shade or two deeper for eyes or lips.

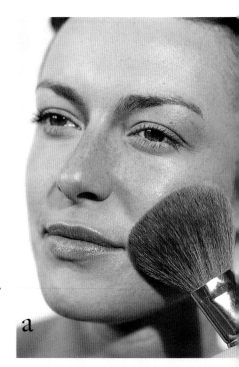

a

1 On fresh, clean skin, spritz your face with a little refreshing rosewater or facial spray. Pat dry, apply a little moisturizer, wait a few minutes, and then touch out blemishes, dark circles and marks with a brush dipped in concealer. Blend the edges, using warm fingertips. Artificial light, unlike the softness of candlelight, can be harsh on shadows around the eyes. So don't miss. If you feel you need foundation on the rest of your skin, then apply it before the concealer, but try to go without for a fresher look.

2 Powder keeps the rest of your make-up in place. Take a large powder brush for a light, sheer finish (as shown, a). Afterwards, use a clean powder puff to press the powder into your skin.

3 To add definition to eyes, prime them first with powder, and then all-over eyeshadow that matches your skin tone. Next apply a contouring eyeshadow (mushroom is a good shade for most skin types) on the upper eyelid with the main emphasis of colour on the outer corner of the lid. Highlight the shape of your browbones with a hint of shimmery powder (as shown, b), and add a touch of pale shimmer to the inner corners of the eyes to brighten them up and make them appear bigger.

4 Eyeliner gives evening make-up the edge. Liquid is quick and handy and gives a very definite line, but it can look harsh. To soften, draw the line in pencil (as shown, c), lining over the top with a liquid or wet shadow/cake liner. Finish with two coats of mascara on the upper lashes, and finally comb through them.

5 Add elegance by elongating the length of your brows. Using a good firm, waxy brow pencil, fill in any sparse areas with upward strokes – follow the arch of your brow up and then carry the tapered end outwards, finishing it just beyond where your brow naturally tapers off.

6 Dramatize your mouth with high-shine glossy lips, but moisturize well first. Apply lip colour straight from the tube. Rich plum suits almost every woman for evening. You don't need to worry about a precise edge as the gloss on top will blur the edges – and lipliner looks unattractive with a full, glossy mouth. Finish with a dab of gloss to the centre of both lips. Work outwards, using a lipbrush (as shown, d) and blending as you go.

7 Choose a powder blusher – it stays in place better than cream. Using a big powder brush, start on the apple of your cheeks and slowly work it outwards, blending it away at the edges.

8 Add shimmer to the tops of your cheekbones. With a powder highlighter, and either your fingertips or a separate brush, place it only on smooth areas of your skin which don't have fine lines, to give a plumper, 'rounded' look.

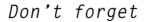
Don't forget

- Keep a tiny book of oil-blotting sheets in your evening bag.
- Carry a tube of clear gloss to add a sexy shine that catches the light, and looks pretty on lips and cheeks.
- Make the skin on your body as appealing as the skin on your face with shimmery highlighting fluids.
- If you are going to wear false eyelashes, use single ones. That way, if they fall out, it's just one that can be innocently brushed away, rather than a whole set.
- Maximize your smile with a tooth-brightening toothpaste.

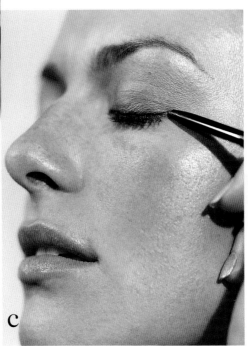

b

c

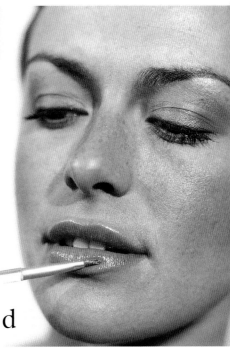

d

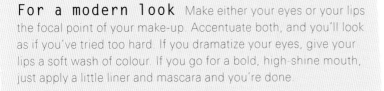

For a modern look Make either your eyes or your lips the focal point of your make-up. Accentuate both, and you'll look as if you've tried too hard. If you dramatize your eyes, give your lips a soft wash of colour. If you go for a bold, high-shine mouth, just apply a little liner and mascara and you're done.

beautifiers

Make-up can perform miracles when you want to play up your best features. Here are four important techniques that help you make the most of what you've got. Set aside 10–20 minutes once a week before your evening facial routine for a little experimentation. Play and perfect.

how to get great-looking skin

COLOUR IS THE HARDEST PART TO GET RIGHT. MOST WOMEN ARE NOT CONFIDENT ABOUT WHAT COLOUR THEIR SKIN IS, OFTEN BELIEVING IT TO BE PINKY WHEN IT IS MORE YELLOW. MAKE THIS YOUR NUMBER ONE RULE: FOUNDATION NEVER ADDS COLOUR TO THE SKIN. IT SHOULD BLEND IN WITH YOUR NATURAL SKIN TONE ALONG THE JAWLINE, NEXT TO THE NECK.

To find the right colour for you, test a shade at the jawline. If it vanishes on your skin, you've found it. Never go darker with colour: it will be impossible to blend and you will be left with a tell-tale tide mark. Always choose a new foundation in natural daylight.

Foundation comes in many different textures, and the best one to use depends on your skin type and the finish you want.

Two-in-one powder foundations (also called cream-to-powder) are speedy, compact formulas that give a matt, dry powdery finish. Great if you're on the run, these are ideal for normal to oily skins, but too drying on dehydrated, mature skins.

Stick foundations are popular, convenient and easy to use – just dot where you need cover. Dry skins suit these least, but provided you prime your skin well beforehand with moisturizer and blend well, they give excellent coverage.

Satin foundations (also called semi-matt or demi-matt) are often liquid foundations that give a natural, light cover and suit almost all skin types. Some contain light-diffusing pigments that reflect the light, giving the illusion of flawless, younger skin. These are ideal for more mature skin types.

Oil-free foundations are usually water based and contain tiny silicone particles to help them stay in place. They are ideal for oilier skin types that want to reduce the look of shiny skin throughout the day.

Moisturizing foundations are perfect for dry or mature skin – to replace that youthful 'dewy' appearance. Alternatively, try a tinted moisturizer, the perfect summer base. This gives a sheer hint of golden colour and subtly evens out the complexion while giving skin everything it might get from a daily moisturizer.

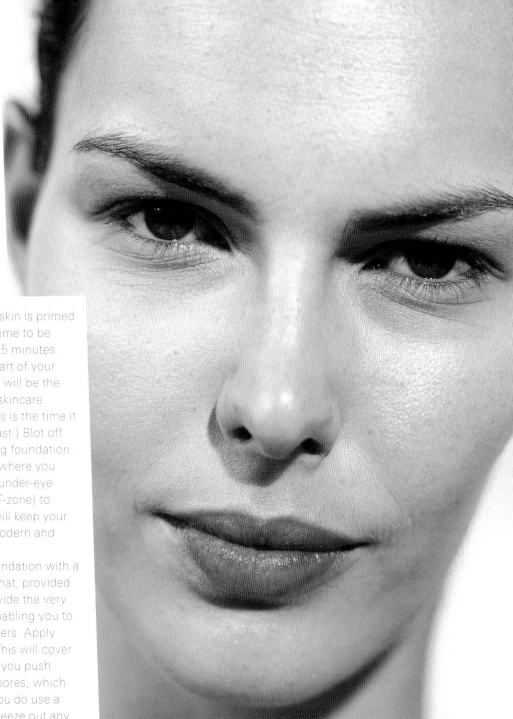

To apply Once your skin is primed with moisturizer, allow it time to be absorbed – it takes up to 15 minutes. (If you make foundation part of your daily regime, moisturizing will be the last part of your morning skincare regime and this 15 minutes is the time it takes to have your breakfast.) Blot off any excess before applying foundation.

Apply foundation only where you need it (on broken veins, under-eye shadows and the central T-zone) to even out skin tone. This will keep your make-up looking fresh, modern and more youthful.

Professionals apply foundation with a sponge. But most agree that, provided they're clean, fingers provide the very best way to do the job, enabling you to blend into the tiniest corners. Apply with downward strokes. This will cover the pores well, otherwise you push pigment up and into the pores, which only highlights them. If you do use a sponge, use it damp. Squeeze out any excess water first and work the foundation into the sponge well so that the application is light and even.

Don't miss Never put too much foundation around the eyes – it will emphasize fine lines and wrinkles. Don't layer bases there either. If you plan to use a concealer around the eye area, don't use foundation. It'll look too heavy and dry.

Remember Apply foundation to your ears, which are often slightly redder than your face. Always work by a window so that you are in natural light. And the experts' secret...blend, blend, blend into your skin.

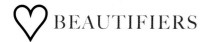

how to enhance your eyes

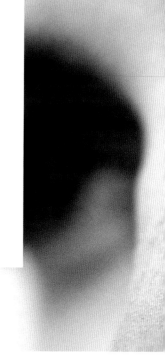

WELL, YOU CAN'T CHANGE THE SHAPE OF YOUR EYES WITHOUT SURGERY, BUT EYESHADOW ALLOWS YOU TO CREATE THE ILLUSION OF BIGGER, WIDER, NARROWER OR DEEPER EYES WITH JUST A LITTLE CLEVER SHADING AND CONTOURING. IT'S ONE OF THE MOST USEFUL ITEMS OF MAKE-UP AT THE BOTTOM OF THE BAG, AND ONE THAT WE RARELY USE TO ITS FULL POTENTIAL.

For the most modern look, keep it simple. A clean sweep of a single colour, matt or shimmery, is all you need for daytime. But experiment a little more for evening or special occasions, using shadows to shape and contour the eyes for more definition or to create a smoky effect. Matts are best for contouring, while iridescent shadows work as highlighter. Use dark shadows to create depth and to make prominent areas recede, and light shadows to emphasize and make less prominent areas stand out.

The basics Avoid putting eye cream on just before you make up or your eyeshadow will crease in seconds. And remember: if eye make-up is going to stay in place, it's important to prime skin properly first so even out your skin tone and cover any tiny bluish veins with foundation, and then use a velour powder puff to pat the eyelids with a little sheer translucent face powder.

Using a matt eyeshadow that perfectly matches your skin tone, blend across the entire area, from lashes to brow, using a shadow brush. Apply any shade or texture of powder eyeshadow you choose on top, and it will blend in a wash of colour you can build up for more intensity or to contour. Dark shadow applied closer to your lashes creates a wonderfully smoky effect – use pencil eyeliner too to softly smudge the finish.

Remember Avoid matching eyeshadow to the colour of your eyes (check your ideal colours on pages 150–1), especially if your eyes are green or blue. Neutral colours that contrast with your eye colour work best.

Quick tips

● Curling your eyelashes (see page 165) makes your eyes look bigger and your lashes longer and neater. So your mascara looks more groomed too.

● If you have blonde eyelashes, get them tinted. Or paint liquid eyeliner (match your mascara) on your lash roots, using a fine brush.

● If you're not wearing much eye make-up, navy mascara makes eyes look more vibrant and sparkling.

● If you find it hard to apply eyeliner, try keeping your elbows steady on a table, look down into a mirror and stretch the skin along the lid before applying.

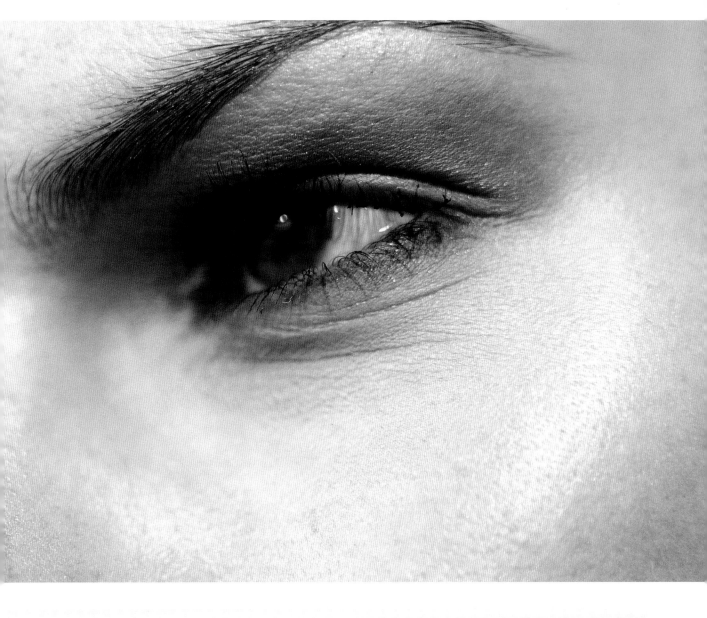

Small eyes Apply a pale eyeshadow over the entire eyelid and up to the browbone, and then add a slightly darker colour in the socket line to emphasize the contour. Now place a little dab of white eyeshadow on the browbone to widen.

Large eyes Stick to the darker, matt shades of eyeshadow. For large eyelids, choose a deeper eye colour, applying over the lid and into the socket, and then blend well.

Wide-set eyes Use a pale shadow over the entire lid and then add a deeper colour in and above the crease on the inner half of the eye. Apply eyeliner all along the upper lid, making it slightly thicker at the inner corner of the eye.

Close-set eyes Apply pale shadow on the inner corner of the lid, and then blend dark shadow on the outer corner. Apply eyeliner along the upper and lower lashline, winging it out at the sides.

Deep-set eyes Stick to pale shades of eyeshadow, such as beige, ivory, champagne and lilac, over the entire eyelid and close to the lashes. Use brown eyeliner on the top lashline only.

Droopy lids Shade the outer corners of the eyes, tapering colour upward and outward (like tiny wings).

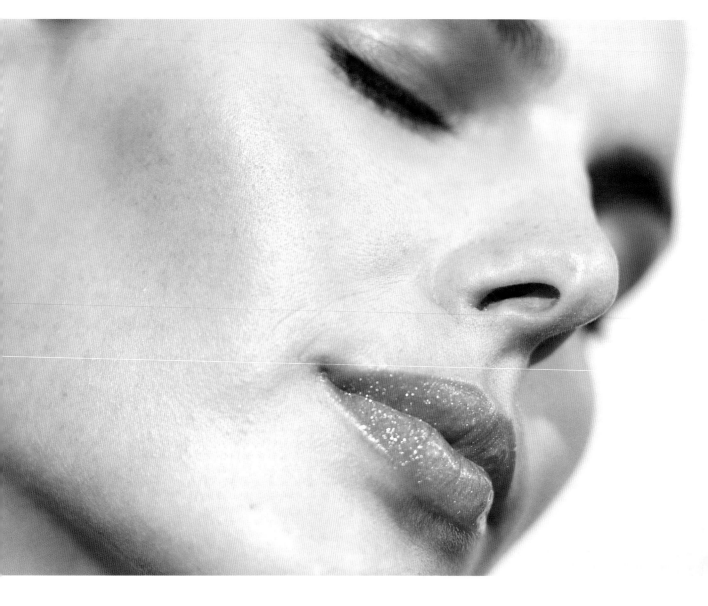

how to reshape your lips

YOU CAN USE LIP COLOUR TO CHANGE THE NATURAL SHAPE OF YOUR MOUTH. BUT KEEP IT SUBTLE. DON'T TRY TO ALTER THE ENTIRE LIPLINE – THE FAKERY JUST LOOKS MORE AND MORE OBVIOUS AS THE COLOUR FADES AWAY.

Corrections are more effective if you use a subdued colour, such as matt medium tones in your natural lip colour. Steer clear of red: it is one of the worst shades to use. It's so bright that it draws attention to the mouth, and shows up a false lip shape.

The basics Block out your natural shape, using concealer or a foundation stick to match the surrounding skin tone. Then practise with lipliner, softly drawing in the shape you want, going inside or outside the natural line. NEVER go too far. Minor adjustments done thoughtfully are far more convincing.

Once you are happy with the shape, it's time to add colour. Avoid a heavy, matt lipline. Keep the new shape undefined and glossy with a shimmery nude shade of lip colour to make your lips appear bigger. Dark colours make lips look thinner. Add a dab of gloss to the centre of the bottom lip to make it appear bigger, rounded and full.

how to shape your cheeks

BLUSHER GIVES YOUR FACE A REAL LIFT AND ADDS A LITTLE COLOUR, BUT DON'T WASTE YOUR TIME TRYING TO CONTOUR IN CHISELLED CHEEKBONES WHERE THERE AREN'T ANY. MAKE-UP ARTISTS ALL AGREE THAT BLUSHER ALWAYS LOOKS BEST ON THE APPLE OF THE CHEEK, WHICH IS WHERE COLOUR WOULD NATURALLY RISE IF YOU WERE EMBARRASSED OR FLUSHED AFTER EXERCISE. HERE IT ALSO MAKES THE FACE LOOK MORE YOUTHFUL (ESPECIALLY ONCE EARLY PLUMPNESS HAS GONE).

Quick tips

● Whatever blusher you choose, make sure it's slightly pink so skin stays looking baby fresh.
● If your blusher looks too bright, soften it by layering a neutral colour (skin-tone face powder is ideal) over the top.
● Always apply blusher as the final step in your make-up routine. The last thing you want to do is overplay its effect by applying too much colour too early on.

The basics Remember: the apple is the round, lifted part of your face that you find by smiling in an exaggerated way. Dust it, using a circular motion. And make sure you blend the colour up into the hairline at the sides.

Round or wide face If your cheekbones are virtually non-existent, place colour on them too. Pick up the tiniest amount of blusher on the brush, dust off the excess and then, starting at the ears, make a semicircular swoosh along the cheekbone, finishing on the apple of the cheek. Repeat a few times to build up the colour. Finally wipe the brush and then sweep it again, this time in the usual direction – from the apple to the ear. It will soften the effect and ensure any fine facial hairs are now lying flat.

Narrow face You need a little shimmery highlighter to give the illusion of width. Apply blusher on the apples of your cheeks as usual – to give the impression of fuller cheeks – and then apply a touch of sheer gloss along the tops of the cheekbones.

High forehead and gaunt temples Apply blusher across the brow close to the hairline. Add to the browbones to give warmth to the eyes at the same time.

Pointed chin or chiselled jaw Soften your features with just a touch of blusher on the chin.

Thin lips Apply a layer of light-reflective concealer all over the lip area and on to the skin. By magically illuminating the whole area, it makes lips appear bigger. But for the quickest lip plump, simply apply a little lip gloss to the centre of your lower lip.

Lip essentials

● To give a softer finish to an older mouth, try outlining your lips *after* applying lipstick. This way it won't stand out and look obvious, but you've still given your lipline more shape.
● Apply lots of lip balm before you go to bed. In the morning your lips will be softer and more supple.

boosters

When you need a little extra loving attention, use these beauty boosters to enhance the rest of your make-up. An elegant brow, a sexy, natural-looking tan, curled lashes and coloured face powders – each adds a finishing touch.

how to reshape your brows

EYEBROWS ARE AN UNDERRATED PART OF THE FACE. EVEN IN REPOSE, THE ARCH, SHAPE AND WIDTH OF YOUR BROWS CREATE AN EXPRESSION ON YOUR FACE, AND THAT INSTANTLY AFFECTS HOW PEOPLE WILL PERCEIVE YOU. NEAT, DEFINED BROWS OPEN UP YOUR EYES AND ENHANCE THEIR SHAPE, MAKING YOU APPEAR WARMER AND MORE RESPONSIVE.

Getting the shape right

1 The brow's thicker, inner edge should start vertically above the inner corner of the eye.

2 To determine the other end, use the old trick of holding a pencil along the side of your nose and then swinging the top of it past the outer corner of your eye – where it touches is where the brow should end. (Brows that extend too far pull eyes down, making them look droopy.)

3 The arch of your brow should be about half way along, just beyond the outer edge of the iris when you look straight ahead.

4 If you are still unsure where to pluck, blank out the hairs where you'd like to see skin, using a white eye pencil. This really helps you get a good idea of the final effect, keeps both brows balanced and reduces the risk of mistakes.

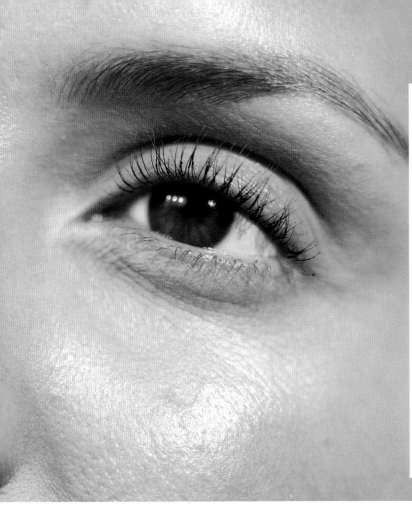

Filling in for emphasis

If your brows are pale, thin or sparse, use a brow pencil that matches their natural colour or is a tone lighter (never darker). Keeping the colour light complements your hair. Filling in is also the interim solution if you've over-plucked in the past and your brows are now too thin – but try to grow them back.

● Draw colour in with tiny, upward, feathery strokes, working in the direction of hair growth, and subtly extend the line at the outer ends.

● If you prefer to use powder, tap off any excess, and apply colour to the arch first. Next go back to the inner end, fill in, blend through and taper off at the other end. Then brush, using a stiff brow brush to work the colour through the brows upward and outward, following your natural browline.

The technique

● Take your time and use a magnifying mirror in daylight.
● Start by tidying up obvious stray hairs – this may be all you need to make a difference.
● Always pluck one hair at a time.
● Pull each hair out with a swift, sharp tug in the direction in which it is growing, while holding the skin around it taut with the other hand as you pull.
● Never shape the top hairs or your brows will end up patchy and unbalanced. However, if the hairs are long (making it hard to keep them neat), you can snip their length a little. Do this only to hairs between the inner brow end (nearest your nose) and the arch – never trim the tapering hairs. Brush them straight upward (with a cleaned-up old mascara wand if you don't have a brow brush), and, taking a small, sharp pair of scissors, snip the tips off the long hairs, always keeping in line with the top of your brow. Finally groom back into shape.
● When changing the shape, do a few hairs on one brow and then some on the other so they balance. Step back regularly to make sure they match and keep checking your progress, using the pencil trick as your guide.

Brow waxing

If you've never been happy with your brows, I'd really recommend a brow wax. It doesn't hurt as much as you might imagine, and the neat skin, free from any little hairs, makes you look extremely groomed. Once you have the desired shape, it's easier to maintain yourself. But brows are high maintenance and a new shape may need attention all week.

Fast track If you find plucking painful, try after a shower or bath. It's the best time because your skin is warmer so the pores are open.

Don't miss Still too painful? Ice your brows first to numb the sensation or use a little anaesthetic baby-teething gel.

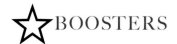
how to camouflage blemishes

BY DAY 14 OF YOUR NUTRITION REGIME THERE SHOULD BE LESS DARKNESS UNDER THE EYES AND A BETTER SKIN TONE. STILL, IT'S GOOD TO KNOW THAT CONCEALER IS THERE FOR OCCASIONAL DARK CIRCLES, THREAD VEINS, SPOTS AND BLEMISHES. SOMETIMES IT'S THE SUBTLE LITTLE THINGS YOU DO THAT MAKE ALL THE DIFFERENCE.

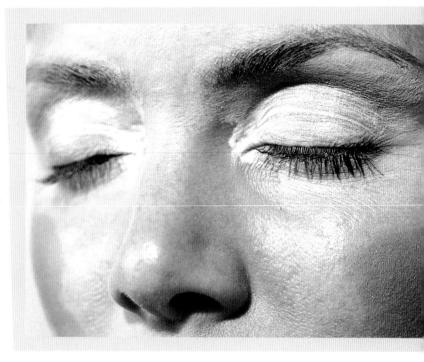

Remember: yellow-based concealer is the best colour for all skin tones. The most common mistake is to use a concealer that is too pale or too pink – these will simply sit on your skin and show up imperfections, rather than blend in. Choose a colour that is one shade lighter than your foundation, if using one. Many make-up artists favour using concealer alone so skin is kept as fresh and natural as possible. Under-eye concealers are thinner and often contain light-diffusing particles that bounce harsh light off dark areas, making them appear brighter

Dark circles Pick up a tiny amount of concealer on your finest brush (see page 146). Hold a mirror at eye level, look ahead and then tilt your chin downward to show the darkness up at its worst. Carefully paint the concealer onto the dark areas only, patting lightly into place.

Eye bags Apply concealer on the area of shadow directly beneath the bags, not on the bags themselves, or you'll be highlighting them.

Don't skimp Keep the brush clean by washing it regularly, especially if you use it to camouflage spots and pimples.

Top tip If you want to cover up patches of redness (such as around the nose or on the cheeks), stick to foundation rather than concealer. Concealer is too light and will highlight rather than hide.

Colour correction

YOU MAY HAVE SEEN GREEN CONCEALER, DESIGNED TO TONE DOWN REDNESS, AND COLOUR CORRECTIVE CONCEALERS ALSO COME IN SEVERAL OTHER COLOURS, INCLUDING APRICOT, PEACH, WHITE AND LILAC – BUT ALL REQUIRE A LIGHT-HANDED APPPROACH. THEY ARE AVAILABLE IN FLUID OR POWDER FORM.

If you want to experiment with a colour-corrective product, blend it with your usual foundation or powder rather than letting it sit on your skin in a separate layer.

Apricot is a radiance booster and an effective pick-me-up for tired, dull skin.

Blue gives pale skin a certain ethereal quality.

Green takes the redness out of spots and blemishes, red thread veins, ruddy cheeks and sunburn. However, red and green make grey so use the tiniest amount.

Lilac revives tired, sallow skin and adds radiance under the glare of harsh lights.

Peach or yellow evens out skin tone and can give the complexion a flattering finish.

White adds luminosity and lightens dark circles under eyes.

Rose or pink gives back that subtle radiance of youthful skin to a tired complexion.

how to fake tan your face

GET THAT GOLDEN GLOW OF SUMMER WITHOUT THE SUN DAMAGE. FAKE TANS ARE BETTER THAN EVER, ESPECIALLY FOR LIGHTER-COLOURED SKIN TONES.

First use a face scrub (see pages 94–5) and then moisturize well and wait for at least 10 minutes for it to be absorbed. Next smear a little petroleum jelly over your brows to avoid colour collecting here. Apply the self-tan to your face, using light, sweeping movements and blending it away before you get to the hairline. Massage in well. Add a little self-tan to the backs of your hands, too, and then wash your palms thoroughly.

Or use a tinted moisturizer Great for spring, when you want to add a bit of healthy radiant colour, these creams are sheer and blend in easily to boost your natural skin tone.

how to curl your lashes

YOU'LL BE AMAZED BY THE DIFFERENCE IT MAKES. CURLED LASHES ADD EMPHASIS AND GIVE THE ILLUSION OF BIGGER, WIDER-OPEN EYES.

Always curl your lashes before you apply mascara or you risk breaking them. Look straight ahead into a mirror and position the curlers around the upper lashes, ensuring that you do not catch any skin. Press down firmly for a count of 10. Then roll the curler upward and away while still holding onto the lashes. Release and repeat on the other eye.

Or try perming your lashes For stubborn, straight lashes, a perm lasts about a month and makes a dramatic difference.

Caught without your lipstick? Rub on a little rosy blusher, or some toffee-coloured shadow, and seal with lip balm.

To make the whites of your eyes appear brighter Use a pale blue pencil under your eyes. Alternatively, soft blue eyeshadow lightly dusted under the eyes works well.

Blobbed your mascara? Use a clean, damp mascara wand to separate clogged lashes, and a damp cotton bud to clean any blobs from the skin.

Tend to get lipstick on your teeth? Place your index finger in your mouth, close your lips around it and pull your finger out. Any lipstick that would have ended up on your teeth comes off on your finger.

Your mascara always smudges? If it still smudges once you've left it off your bottom lashes, try wearing a waterproof version (but these are hard to remove).

In a rush? Apply a neutral, pinky-brown lip colour rather than red or other deep-coloured lipsticks which require more precise application.

fast track

Tired skin? Wear an apricot-coloured blusher to make it look more radiant. And add a little suble shimmer to give cheeks a soft, more rounded effect.

For a softer eyeline on mature skin Use shadow along the lashline rather than pencil or liquid. It's easier to control too.

Applying powder around the mouth Blow out your cheeks as you apply so less powder collects in the creases.

Retouching make-up during the day? Spritz your face with a facial mist first. This will dampen the make-up (making it easier to blend), give your skin a boost and help to soften fine lines.

Run out of concealer? Use the dry residue around the neck of your foundation bottle. It's thicker, like the texture of most concealers, and should match your skin tone perfectly too.

If your concealer makes your eyes appear crepey or baggy The texture is probably too heavy. And, if your skin is also dry, you may need to apply eye cream first. Apply only a little and make sure that it is well absorbed (ideally with a matt finish) so concealer looks smooth applied on top.

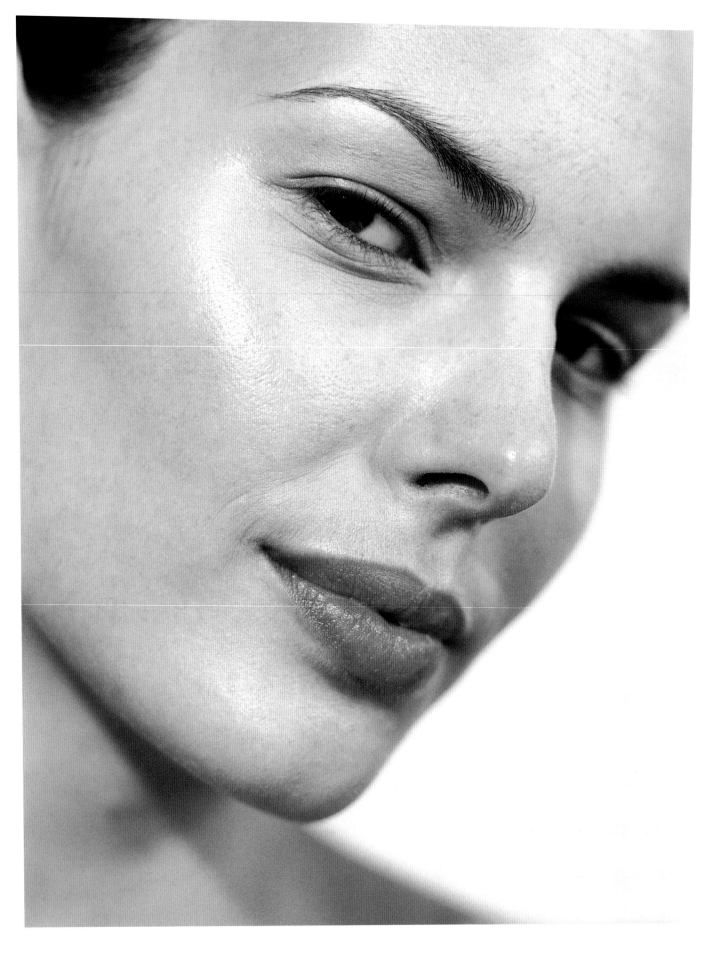

keeping it going

Declutter your make-up bag

Throw away anything that's been in your make-up bag for up to three years. (Include dried-up mascaras, colour palettes you never use and lipsticks which you 'might wear one day'.) You're ready to start afresh.

Re-invent yourself

Colour psychologists believe that the colours you wear can dramatically change the way you feel as much as the way you look. That applies to lipsticks, too – especially red lipsticks. Red lipstick is all about power and strength. It's the colour of energy and seduction. From a psychologist's point of view, if you wear red you're either very lively, or you'd like to be. Either way, red demands attention. It is exciting, assertive, dynamic and passionate, but at the same time it is a rather good colour to hide behind, so choose it when you feel sluggish, too, to give the impression of having more energy than you feel. Brunettes and those with olive or black skins suit red best, but anyone can wear a red lipstick sometimes – yes, even redheads – provided it's applied carefully and isn't competing with heavy eye make-up.

Go make-up shopping

Ask for help at make-up counters if you feel overwhelmed by choice. Choose a store you trust and a brand you like the look of and try something new. Don't just grab the colours that attract you and make a dash for the sales till. Subtle classic colours don't always stand out on the counter. Seek advice from a friend (for extra support and more fun) or from classic, understated brands. It's almost impossible to be objective about what really suits you, so expert guidance can help you avoid expensive mistakes.

Put on a happy face

Make-up to feel good. Even when you're feeling down, just making the effort to 'put on your face' can provide a much-needed lift and boost the spirits.

Practise

Stick with something simple, such as the fast track make-up regime if you haven't worn make-up regularly for years. Get into the habit of applying it without fail each morning on a freshly cleansed and moisturized face and you'll soon be used to the feeling of being groomed. It takes less time than you think to bring out the best in your face. You may be amazed at the effect it has on others, too – how you look has a lot to do with the way people relate to you. You're simply more appealing.

Stay out of that rut

Plan a big night out or arrange a party every two to four weeks – something that requires a little more effort in the make-up department. The effort it will take will keep you on your toes. (Turn to page 244 for the hot-date programme – a hot date can, of course, be with your husband or girlfriends.) The rule is: never go on a night out without adding some sort of sparkle to your make-up, whether it's a highlighter shadow on your eyes or a shimmering body powder lightly dusted over your shoulders.

Invest in a make-up lesson

An experienced make-up artist will teach you other new tricks. Either go to the counter of a make-up brand you like or contact a make-up artist direct through a hair and make-up agency. Or try ringing your favourite magazine for local recommendations.

Rules for everyday grooming

● Avoid too much shine by always carrying a little book of powdered papers. Impregnated with a fine layer of powder, they will blot excess oil.

● Vow never to let your eyebrows grow straggly again – check them over every couple of days.

● Always, always remove your make-up before bed, no matter how tired you are. You'll feel much better, and your skin will thank you. If you don't, you'll wake up with clogged pores and smudged eyes.

Don't be fashion's slave

Make-up trends change so fast these days that you barely have time to catch on to a new thing before it's gone. In the past, we could stick with a look for a decade (think '50s eyeliner, followed by the '60s passion for creamy frosted eyeshadow) and still get away with being stylish and 'modern'. Now, no sooner has lilac become trendy than blue is back, and gold is waiting for its magical 'modern' moment.

What we all seem to forget while trying to keep up is what actually suits us: our individual colouring and lifestyle demands. Sure, sometimes something amazing comes along (such as those fabulous all-in-one eye, lip and cheek sticks) and becomes a firm favourite in your make-up bag, but never lose sight of you. The art of perfecting you and you alone is what make-up is for. If you must follow fashion, then change the colour of your nail polish daily, revamp your lip colour, but otherwise leave everything else to the teens – you just don't need it any more.

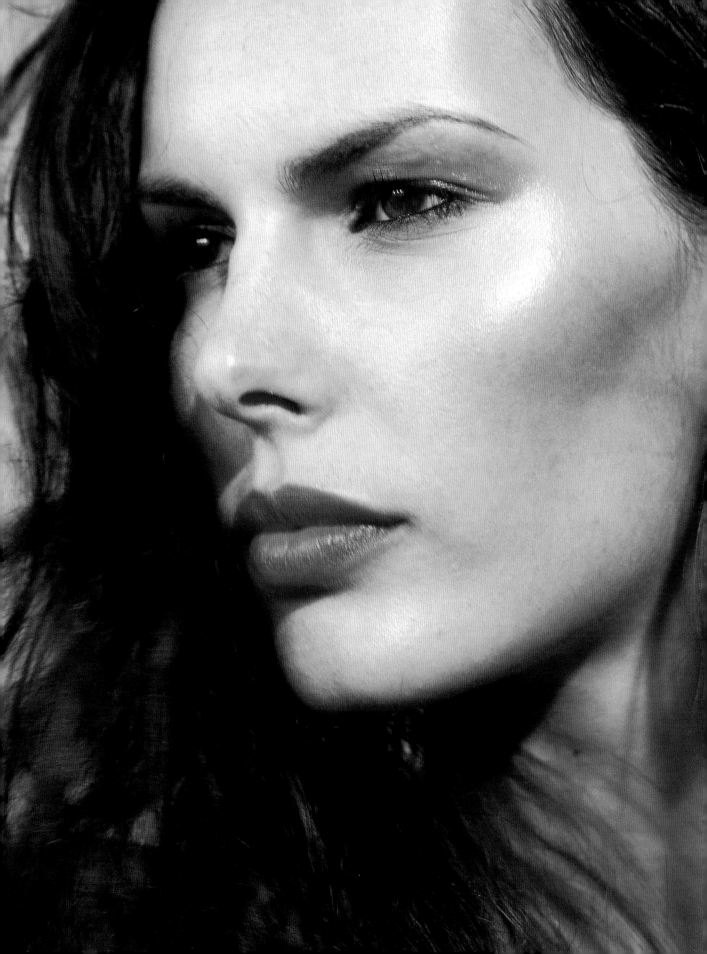

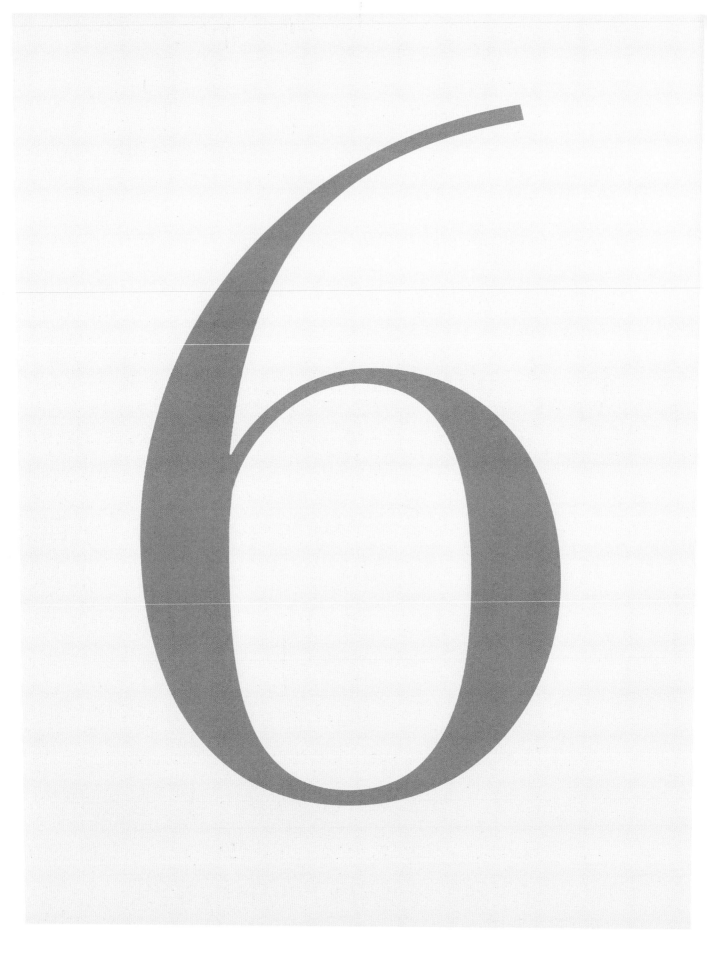

21 DAYS

TO

GLOSSY

HAIR

Discover fresh confidence as you express yourself through your outer beauty. Soft, silky and shining - let your hair reflect that new-found radiance.

Your haircare
programme

This programme aims above all to bring the condition and shine back into your hair. To achieve the kind of glossy, groomed, glamorous hair you always admire on others. By boosting your haircare regime, along with your Nutrition and Relaxed Living programmes, you'll come to understand and appreciate your hair a little more, manage it much better, and have a clearer idea of what it needs from a style when you're at the hairdresser.

YOUR HAIR SAYS MORE ABOUT YOUR HEALTH AND THE WAY YOU CARE FOR YOURSELF THAN PERHAPS YOU REALIZE.

Hair as statement Always on show, much like your face, your hair is a clear expression of your personality. If it looks shiny, well cared for and stylish, it can make you look and feel so good it almost doesn't matter what you're wearing. And, of course, the opposite is true. So this 21-day regime is all about getting the most from your hair with ease. It incorporates all the best advice on the right products for your hair type, plus how to blow-dry with confidence, sort out your colour and get your hair back into shape with the most flattering cut for your face. Can't wait to see it...

What do I need to change? Poor diet (too many dairy foods, excess alcohol, especially white wine, vitamin B and iron deficiency), intense blow-drying, chemical processing (that means colouring and perming) and stress – all take their toll on the quality of your hair. Not to mention years under attack from the elements (UV exposure, wind and seawater), pollution and chlorine. Sure, you cut it and it grows again, but mistreated hair becomes weak, especially when coupled with prolonged illness and hormonal fluctuations. Split ends are an obvious symptom of hair that has grown brittle, fine and less flexible.

Remember Like your skin, you need to feed your hair, from the inside out...and the outside in.

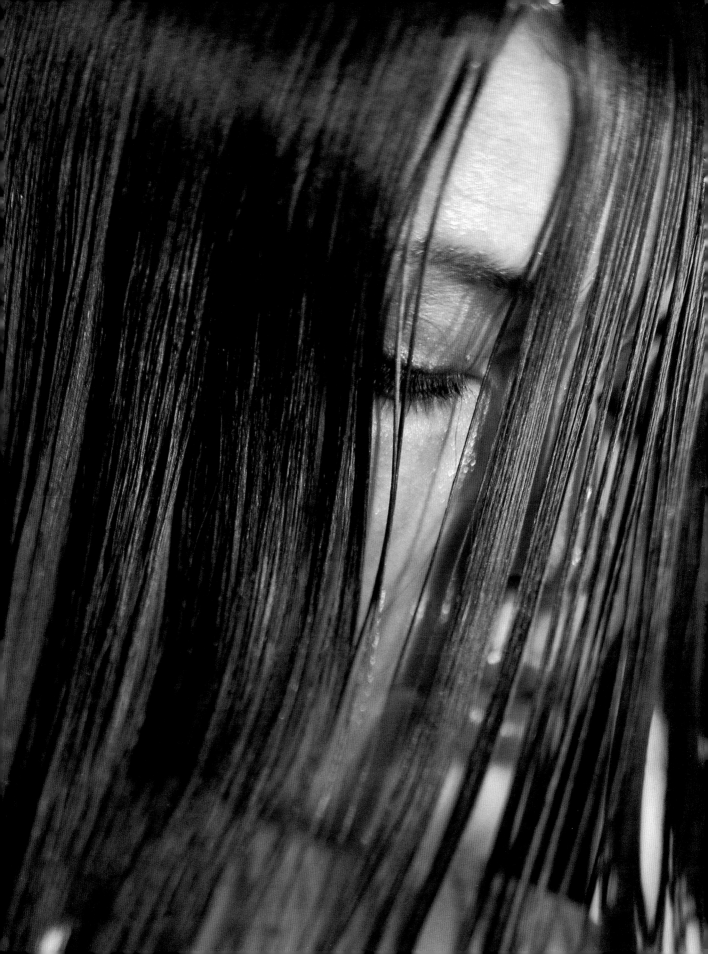

What you do in these 21 days

if you're 20-35...

Your hair is still flexible and supple, and if you're not into colour you may well still have nearly 100 per cent of your natural colouring, so build on your assets. But daily experiment may be putting your hair under constant physical abuse as fashion trends for colour and intensive styling, such as straightening irons or crimpers, come and go. And you may also be under stress from work and relationships, while poor nutrition is no better for your hair than it is for your body.

● Condition to protect your hair from styling. Conditioning also protects from the elements.
● Improve your cleansing technique to help with scalp problems and remove residue from styling products.
● Protect your hair in the sun on holidays as you would your face. A two-week holiday can severely frazzle your hair.
● Avoid dieting. Poor nutrition is believed to be the number one reason for hair problems in young women. You need plenty of oily fish (rich in omega-3 oil) and vitamin-B-rich dark green vegetables for great-looking hair. Look back over your Nutrition programme now.

...35-50

You may still have at least 50 per cent of your natural colour. However, styling will have affected the condition of your hair, making it feel finer and more brittle. It's not too late to take action. You can start by making your hair feel softer and look more nourished and shiny. And in these mid-years you should try to reduce any stress in your life.

● Incorporate hair beautifying treatments, such as a perfect blow-dry. Pamper your hair with a weekly intensive conditioning treatment – it's great for hair that's coloured too.
● After week two, find a new cut that flatters your softer features and better conditioned hair.
● Add scalp massage to your regime, either when you shampoo or as a once-a-week intensive treatment. Make time for relaxation techniques (see chapter 7) to reduce stress.
● Keep up your Nutrition programme.

...50 and over

Hormonal changes mean that your hair may feel much drier, making it less flexible, even brittle, and more prone to splitting. Pamper it all the more.

● Yes, it's moisturize, moisturize, moisturize. Conditioner will help to keep it supple and less prone to breakage. Treat yourself to the conditioning hair mask, and try using leave-in conditioners.
● Use serums to smooth dry, rough cuticles (see page 183) and thickening products to fatten each hair strand as hair gets fine.
● Trim regularly. It keeps your hair more manageable and will avoid split ends.
● Bump up on protein intake (see chapter 1) for stronger, more resilient hair.

What you'll achieve

Happy hair You see results quickly: great-looking hair that's in the best condition ever. Hair responds well to a lot of love. By stepping up your haircare, along with back-up from the Nutrition and Low-Stress programmes, your scalp will be much healthier and that means shinier, more manageable hair.

Low-maintenance hair At the end of this programme, you will have a much clearer idea of what your hair needs. And, I hope, you'll have begun to live with your hair the way it is and to work with it, rather than trying to change it against its will. The aim is low-maintenance hair, which is all many of us have time for. It's far better for your hair in the long run to go with its natural texture. And guess what? Experts believe that the hair texture you're born with is the one that truly suits you best. So just accept who you are and accept your hair into the bargain. Make the most of it, of course, enjoy it – it says so much about you – but most of all aim to make it easy.

Empowerment Let's face it – when your hair looks good, you feel wonderful. And a confident toss of the hair is very, very sexy. Think how good you feel when you've spent time and money at the hairdresser (OK, not the money perhaps). With a little effort, you'll be able to create that uplifting feeling for yourself. It's great knowing your hair can look as good as that any time you want. All it takes is a little know-how and practice.

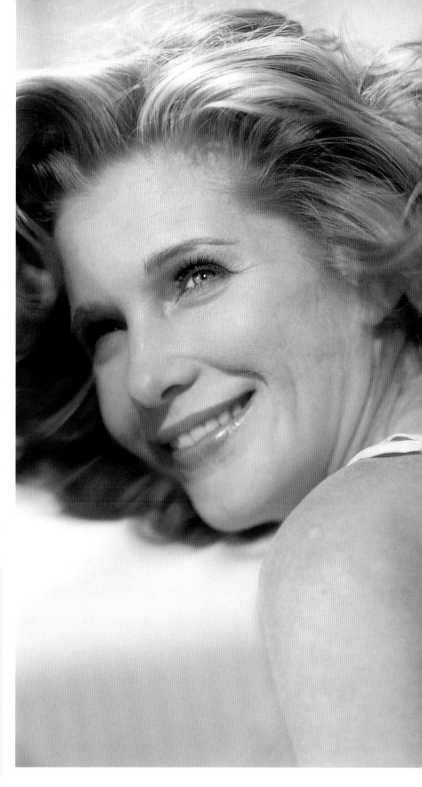

your haircare kit

ALL THE ITEMS REQUIRED FOR THE MUST-DO
DAILY TRANSFORMERS ARE LISTED. ONCE
YOU'VE DECIDED WHICH BEAUTIFIERS AND
BOOSTERS MOST APPEAL TO YOU, PREPARE A
PERSONAL CHECKLIST OF OTHER ESSENTIALS
YOU'LL NEED, SO YOU HAVE EVERYTHING TO
HAND WHEN YOU MOST NEED IT.

Comb

It's vital to disperse conditioner evenly
through the hair and to help gently detangle
without stretching and snapping it. Choose
a 'saw-cut' comb, made from one piece of
wood, metal or plastic, it has no rough
edges to snag hairs.

Comb-grips and large hair-grips

These keep your hair out of the way while
you blow-dry. Choose good-quality ones
that can hold large quantities of hair.

Conditioner

To smooth and soften your hair, choose
conditioner according to the texture of your
hair. Rich and leave-in conditioners are
suitable for very dry or long hair, and
lightweight conditioners for normal hair
that's medium length or short.

Hairdryer

Look around for a model that's lightweight
and really easy to handle, with a cool-air
button, varied speeds and a diffuser
attachment to help emphasize natural curls.
Your hair type determines the wattage: use
a 1500w dryer for fine hair, and 1600–1800w
for thick hair.

Hairspray

This is a fine finishing spray that keeps hair
in place after styling. All styles benefit from
using a little, but limit its use if you have dry
hair as its alcohol content can be drying.

Mousse

It gives body and shape to most hairstyles,
and especially suits fine or lank hair that
needs volume without stickiness.

Pomade

This gives soft styling and texture to layered hair without stickiness and is the modern alternative to wax, which was heavy on the hair and therefore difficult to apply. Great for short, thick hair (curly or straight) and unruly grey hair, it smooths and slicks, adding definition and shine.

Radial brush

Also called a round brush, its medium-length natural bristles grip hair well so it's the perfect blow-dry brush and can be used to smooth, straighten and wave hair. The larger the head (of the brush), the straighter it will make your hair; the smaller the head, the tighter the curl.

Shampoo

Cleanse your hair with a shampoo that matches the condition of the skin on your scalp, whether dry, oily or normal. Use specific shampoos, such as those to detox or swim-shampoos that de-chlorinate hair, to suit the life you lead.

Not everyone needs these, but, if you find them appealing, you probably do

Blow-dry cream Use it either just before or after blow-drying to calm down 'fluffy hair'. It's a cream that looks and feels like a leave-in conditioner, and helps to replenish moisture lost to the hairdryer, making it perfect for normal to dry hair.

Ceramic straightening irons Their flat plates press together to flatten hair and smooth out unwanted kinks. They are great for styles which need poker-straight hair, but limit use to special occasions and keep them moving to minimize heat damage.

Large Velcro® rollers You'll want them for fine, flat hair that needs volume at the roots, or to smooth hair after blow-drying.

Serum (or hair polish or glaze). Usually a silicone-based liquid, it forms a fine film on each hair to help smooth and seal dry ends, calm frizziness and combat static. Serum leaves hair phenomenally shiny and healthy looking. Keep it away from your scalp.

Setting lotion This styling liquid dries to 'set' hair in place, and is used particularly for root hold and when drying hair into a style.

transformers

Wash daily, you say? According to trichologists, if your hair is very short, fine, thin or oily, you live in a city or exercise regularly, then yes. Otherwise every 48 hours is enough. Many scalp or styling problems can be resolved with better, regular cleansing, using a mild frequent-use shampoo. So identify your hair type and care for it to get your hair and scalp in best condition.

cleansing

CLEAN HAIR IS SHINY HAIR. SO WASH IT FREQUENTLY AND, MORE IMPORTANTLY, THOROUGHLY, AND YOU'LL SOON FIND THAT STYLING BECOMES MUCH EASIER. THIS IS BECAUSE NOW YOU ARE REGULARLY GETTING RID OF THE BUILD-UP OF STYLING PRODUCTS THAT ATTRACTED DIRT AND WAS DRYING TO YOUR HAIR.

Dilute your shampoo with water before applying it to your hair to make it milder. Over-shampooing can remove essential moisture by stripping out the hair's natural oils.

To **wash hair properly**, use clear running water and, if you thoroughly wet your hair first, it will need less shampoo to get it clean – just a blob about 2cm (⁄in) across. Concentrate solely on your scalp for the single application of shampoo. The suds should clean the hair itself as you rinse them away. If you are prone to a dry 'dandruff' scalp (much of which is dried styling product left in the hair), make sure that you rinse extremely thoroughly every time.

A final **rinse of cool water** encourages the cuticles of your hair to lie flat before drying. But keep just enough away from your scalp to avoid a chilling shock.

Fast track Before shampooing, add conditioner to the ends of long hair. It will act as a detangler while you wash.

Remember If you are now swimming more frequently as part of your Fitness programme, don't forget you'll need to switch to a de-chlorinating formula. This will protect your hair from the oxidizing effect of the pool water, especially if you are outdoors, where UV light will increase the bleaching effect of chlorine.

Don't miss Poor rinsing is a common reason for dull hair and itchy dry scalps. Wash combs and brushes once a week.

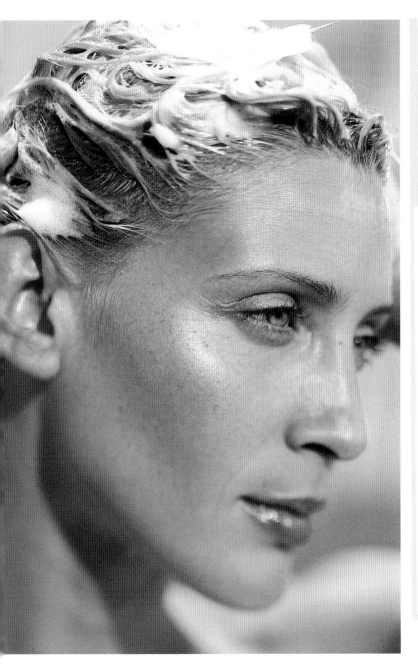

conditioning

CONDITIONING YOUR HAIR EVERY TIME YOU SHAMPOO NOT ONLY SMOOTHS AND SEALS THE OUTER CUTICLE, IT PROVIDES DAILY PROTECTION FROM ENVIRONMENTAL DAMAGE. SO THINK OF CONDITIONER AS A REGULAR MOISTURIZER FOR YOUR HAIR.

All hair needs conditioner to some extent, even lank, oily hair. You just need to choose the right weight for the state of your hair ends, deciding whether they are dry, dull or normal.

Remembering that conditioner is never intended for your scalp, apply midway down your hair if it's normal to dry and not especially fine. Always massage it through to distribute well, and then comb (using a wide-toothed comb) to coat each strand as much as possible. If your hair is fine or oily, you should massage only into the very tips.

Leave-in conditioner is ideal for those with dry hair, afro hair or dry ends.

Intensive conditioner acts like a weekly mask, and not only smooths and seals the cuticle shut, but also gives better protection from both your hairdryer and the weather.

Don't rush your conditioner. Leave it on for the length of time stated on the pack, preferably 2 minutes longer (which feels like ages while you're standing around with wet hair) if your hair is very long and dry. Rinse thoroughly in cool running water.

Don't skimp Only ever comb wet hair. Never brush or it will stretch beyond its elasticity, resulting in snags and splits.

CHOOSE SHAMPOO TO SUIT YOUR SCALP AND CONDITIONER TO SUIT YOUR HAIR, ESPECIALLY IF YOUR SCALP TENDS TO BE EITHER EXCESSIVELY DRY OR OILY. FOR WHILE YOU NEED TO CLEAN AN OILY SCALP AND MOISTURIZE A DRY ONE, HAIR ITSELF HAS FEW OILS. HAIR TEXTURE AND LENGTH SHOULD DICTATE WHICH CONDITIONER YOU NEED, NOT YOUR SCALP.

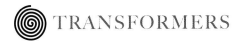 TRANSFORMERS

take-it-easy styling

Learn to love your hair the way it is, going low maintenance with styling skills you can achieve at home. You don't need a shelf load of gear. It's simple. Just know your hair type, the right way to care for it, and the one or two key products that make styling so much easier.

See styling for great-looking, easy-care hair as an essential. You long for straight, straight hair? Do it. Go straight, but wear it curly at least three-quarters of the time if that's what comes naturally. Or if your hair's straight, curl it for fun, but keep it glossy and straight at other times. Pamper your hair, give it the attention it needs, and you'll learn to appreciate it the way it is.

Don't think flat – think smooth and shiny Women with fine hair usually think a perm is the only answer because all they see is that it's too flat. But fine hair shines like no other hair type, especially if you give it a smooth cut.

Don't deny your curls – you've got great body Often those of us with very curly hair want to achieve a more groomed, polished look. But it's worth remembering that natural curls have more body and life than anything you'd ever get from a perm. Separate and smooth the curls with a little serum, and then leave your hair to air dry. If it's long, scoop bits back – pre-Raphaelite style – for easy, desirable hair.

Don't say thick – say volume Avoid thinning out hair that's dense: just appreciate that you have the fullness and body everyone else is desperate to achieve. Get softer, graduated layers and blow-dry, using a little setting lotion to smooth.

Love its natural texture Coarse and wiry? Well, you've got the kind of fullness and body that won't go flat if you get a stylishly layered cut. Baby fine? Bob it into shape and you've got swingy, shiny enviable hair.

Just take a step back and assess your hair – its condition, its style and its colour. What's it really like? What do you like about it? What don't you like about it? One (or more) of the statements below will be you. Take what tips you need and incorporate them into your daily hair regime.

Your hair's looking dull
For smooth, shiny hair, go to 1 (see page 185)

You have dry, split ends
For better condition, go to 3 (see page 186)

Your hair's flat or greasy
For more volume, go to 2 (see page 185)

Your hair's unmanageable
To get control, go to 4 (see page 186)

Don't skimp

Update your shampoo and conditoner. These days you'll find all the latest skincare ingredients in your haircare. Antioxidant vitamins C and E will help to protect against the oxidization which fades hair colour fast. UVA and UVB filters prevent dehydration, splitting and breakage from ultraviolet exposure. Enzymes and AHAs in shampoos help to cleanse hair deep down to remove product build-up and leave hair shiny. And proteins (such as keratin) and amino-acid complexes help to smooth, strengthen and 'rebuild' cuticles (see below).

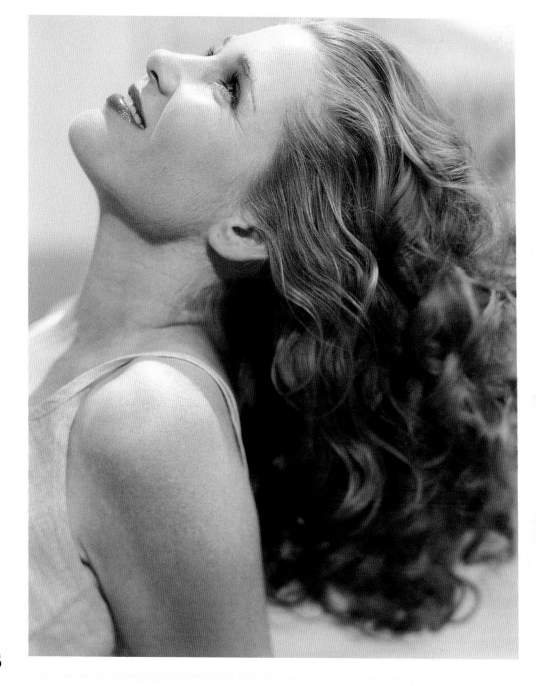

hair facts

● Hair grows from follicles (specialized sacs deep in the skin's lowest layer) and is nourished by its own blood supply.

● Hair cells move upward as they mature (in 21 to 28 days). As they move further from their source of nourishment in the follicle, they turn into the lifeless protein known as keratin. The visible, outermost layer of each hair shaft, called the cuticle, is constantly shedding old, dead keratin cells, in just the same way as the surface of our skin or epidermis sheds dead skin.

● All cell division slows down in your mid-thirties and at this time a number of hair follicles become inactive; by the time you reach your fifties, the number may well have halved.

● Growth rate is controlled by your body's hormones. In women, oestrogen prevents hair growing on the face and diverts it to the rest of the head. Generally we benefit more from this at a younger age (especially during puberty and pregnancy), with thicker, more lustrous hair than men. However, when oestrogen levels drop significantly after the menopause (and after giving birth), hair often becomes thinner and many women may begin to experience some hair loss.

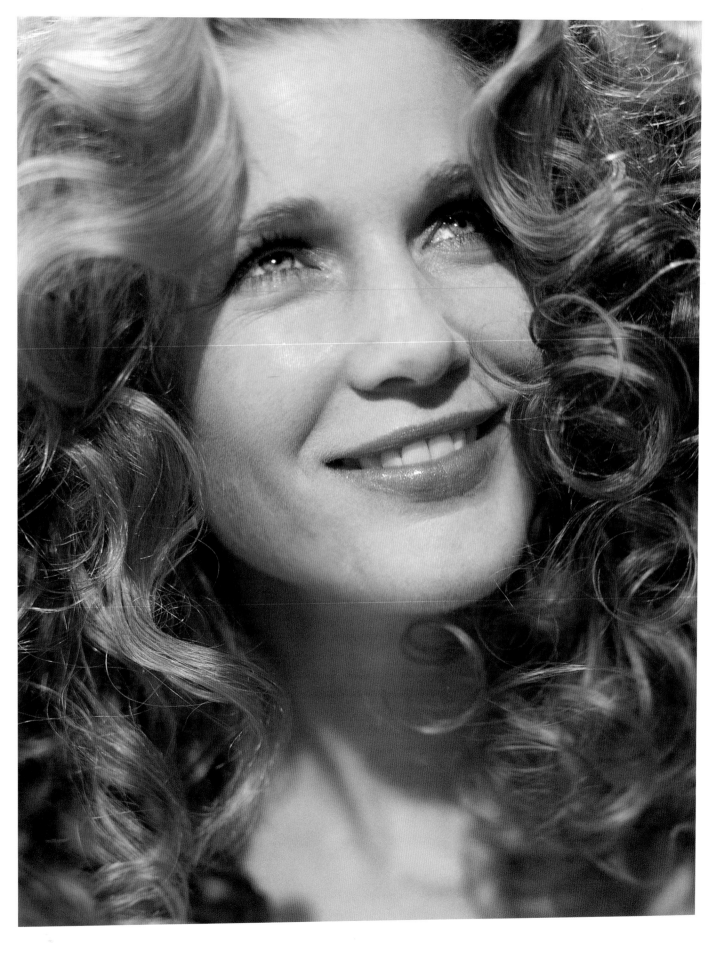

1 to get shine

Hair only looks shiny when the protective coating or cuticle of each hair shaft lies flat, creating a smooth surface that reflects light beautifully. When cuticles become rough through overprocessing (or styling), overheating and poor conditioning, hair looks dull and out of condition.

Clean hair is shiny hair, remember. Oily, city hair needs washing often, due to pollution and dust. And styling products lead to build-up that leaves hair looking dull, too. If you regularly use a range of styling (especially silicone-based) products, you need a deep-cleansing detoxifying shampoo designed to eliminate build-up once a week.

Switch shampoo It refreshes your hair every time you swap because it cleans differently, removing a different level of product build-up.

Deep-conditioning treatments can restore shine by smoothing and sealing the outer cuticle. Try a regular hot-oil treatment for hair past shoulder length – you can do it yourself. Just warm up a half a cup of olive oil, comb through your hair and leave for 5 minutes before shampooing, rinsing thoroughly and then conditioning in the normal way.

Straight hair is shinier than curly hair because smooth hair reflects the light, whereas curls absorb it. Dry hair smooth, using a radial brush to grip the hair well and give more control. Keep the hairdyer nozzle pointing down the hair shaft all the time you are drying, to ensure hair cuticles remain flat. Try setting wavy hair on Velcro® rollers for a smoother finish.

Shine serums and sprays are silicone based to add incredible shine and gloss by varnishing your hair to reflect more light. Apply to towel-dried hair and add a little bit more after styling (once dry) for extra shine. But don't go overboard. If you use more than a couple of drops, hair will instantly become limp, heavy and greasy looking – and you'll be back to square one.

Colour adds shine The warmer your hair colour, the shinier it will look. Brunettes and auburn hair look shinier than blonde or grey hair so add rich – gold or red – highlights.

2 to pump up the volume

Hair that often looks flat, limp, lank or even greasy soon after washing is thin and lacks body at the roots.

Add body with a shampoo and set under a hooded hairdryer. The process of going from wet to dry, hot to cold, under the hood, with your hair on big rollers literally 'sets' it, giving great lift at the roots.

Thin hair tends to be greasy, and generally needs washing every day. Use a mild, frequent-use shampoo.

Avoid 2-in-1 shampoo and conditioners, also called moisturizing shampoos, which leave a residue in the hair that only weighs it down more.

Apply a lightweight conditioner on the ends only if your hair is mid-length to long.

Dry the roots first, parting your hair in sections, and drying it in the opposite direction to which it falls. Give it a final blow-dry with your head upside down.

Volumizing shampoos coat hair to make it look and feel thicker by increasing the diameter of each hair. Root-lift products are mostly spray gels that dry in place, making your roots more rigid.

Style with mousse. Best for fine, lank hair, it's light enough not to weigh hair down. Massage a little into the roots before blow-drying to get lift. To add body, apply further down, comb through and style.

Colour thickens hair Semi-permanent and permanent dyes swell the hair shaft, so hair really is thicker (see page 192).

3 to cope with dry ends

Mainly caused by over-zealous shampooing, not enough conditioner, harsh brushing, and too many heated styling appliances – poor conditioned hair with dry, split ends is largely self-inflicted. However, diet, stress and ill health are major factors too.

Avoid washing dry hair every day: it doesn't need it. And when you do wash, remember to dilute your shampoo. Using less detergent is inevitably less drying. Use heavier, moisturizing shampoos which will leave a fine film of conditioner on the strands. Remember: there is never any need to apply shampoo on the ends – the action of rinsing will be sufficient to cleanse along the whole length of your hair.

Always use conditioner when you shampoo and apply just to the ends, avoiding the roots which may be oilier. Comb to spread evenly. A conditioning mask (see page 191) once a week for 21 days will keep hair softer, supple and easier to style.

Gently remove tangles Tugging and pulling causes breakage and split ends. Your conditioner should also act as a detangler. However, a separate detangling spray may be a solution.

Dry your hair naturally after every other shampoo (or more often), as this will help to lock moisture in rather than drying it out. If you prefer to blow-dry, always keep the hairdryer moving around, and the nozzle at least 15cm (6in) – preferably 30cm (12in) – away from your hair. And remember to angle heat down the hair shaft to ensure that the cuticles lie flat, using the coolest heat possible.

Regularly trim dry, split ends. The thicker, blunt ends make hair look healthier, and your hair is also less likely to split with regular trimming.

Smoothing silicone serums temporarily seal split ends, but these can be hard to wash out and nothing beats a trim.

Vitamin E can nourish dry, brittle hair from within. Eat more nuts and dark green vegetables, and take a daily vitamin E oil capsule.

4 to get control

Frizzy, flyaway hair tends to be quite porous because the hair's natural protection is weak or damaged. It lacks natural moisture so it tends to look worse in rainy or humid weather.

Choose heavier shampoos that contain proteins to coat each shaft, making your hair more supple and helping to tame it down. Rinse thoroughly.

Leave-in conditioner contains anti-humectants (water repellents) which seal the cuticles to prevent moisture from getting into the hair shaft. These can weigh hair down (so take it easy if your hair is fine).

Control frizz by leaving your hair to dry naturally with a serum or pomade massaged in while damp, or cool dry it in sections, starting with the under layers.

Apply styling products evenly through your hair. Whether you choose serum or pomade, the trick is to warm the product in your hands first. Apply to the under layers too – not just to the surface.

Avoid perming frizzy hair; the process can make hair even harder to control afterwards.

Before swimming, apply a conditioner to your hair – any will do – to act as a protective layer from the drying and bleaching effects of chlorine.

Smoothing pomade or serum is essentially a cheat but carry one around with you and apply as often as you think your hair needs calming down. These products will help to seal the cuticle and keep out excess moisture.

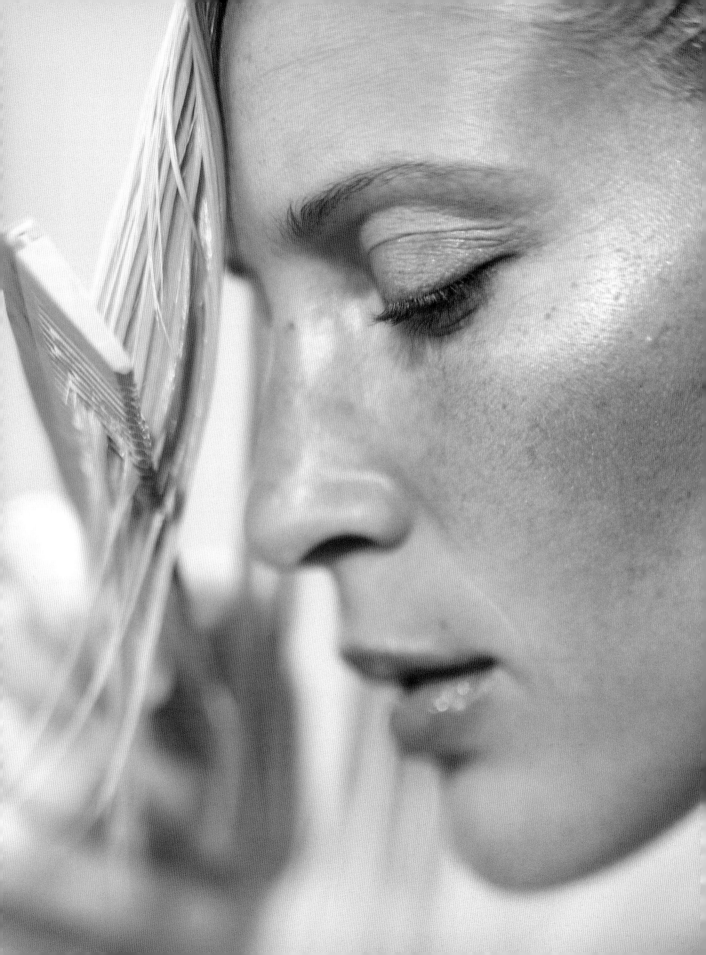

beautifiers

Find time for simple routines and instant know-how tricks that make styling easier so hair looks and feels fabulous every day. Better still, they're the ultimate pampering hair and scalp treatments to soothe and shine.

The perfect blow-dry

BLOW-DRYING IS A PAIN. YOU SPEND AGES DOING IT, AND GIVE UP BEFORE IT'S TOTALLY DRY IF ONLY BECAUSE YOU CAN'T KEEP YOUR ARM IN THE AIR FOR THAT LONG. THEN YOU'RE DISAPPOINTED WITH THE RESULTS: THE SHAPE DOESN'T LAST, AND UNWANTED FRIZZINESS AND KINKS COME BACK THE MOMENT YOU STEP OUTSIDE. BUT MANAGE IT BETTER, AND YOU CAN HAVE THE KIND OF GLOSSY, GROOMED, GLAMOROUS HAIR YOU SEE ON OTHERS.

1 Towel dry your hair all over, and then rough dry with your hairdryer (as shown, a) until it's about 80 per cent dry. Avoid blow-drying hair from soaking wet: not only will it take too long but more heat = more damage. It can stretch hairs until they snap.

2 Apply a small 'ball' of mousse to help control any flyaway tendency, or a blow-dry cream that calms down that fluffy, blow-dried look. Spread between the palms of your hands and apply evenly throughout your hair from the roots. Comb through.

3 Divide your hair into sections (back, front, left side and right side if very long), using comb grips.

4 Start by working at the back, near the nape of the neck, drying the under layers first. This area supports your style, and leaving the top, vulnerable layers until last helps prevent them from drying out. Brush the back section from root to tip, separating it still further, so you only ever dry small sections (as shown, b). This ensures that your hair really is dry.

5 If you are blow-drying smooth and as straight as possible, roll your hair around a large natural-bristle radial brush which holds hair better so you get more control. Pull taut and, with the dryer in your other hand, aim the nozzle down the hair shaft (working from roots to ends) to close and smooth the cuticle as you dry (as shown, c). A flat nozzle attachment on your hairdryer helps you to aim the heat precisely.

6 Work around your head, drying the under-sections first and leaving the front section until last. Dry each section thoroughly before going on to the next.

7 Rub a little shine serum (or blow-dry cream for dry hair) between your fingertips and apply to the ends of your hair to weigh it down (as shown, d) and reduce fluffiness, and then smooth the rest over the surface.

I wouldn't be without a hot-air styling brush. A good all-in-one hot brush and hairdryer has a radial brush head with bristles and is powerful enough to dry hair smoothly as you brush through.

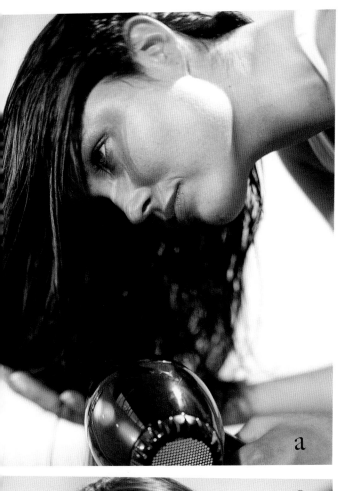

a

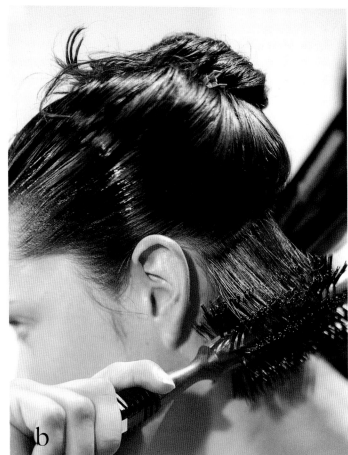

b

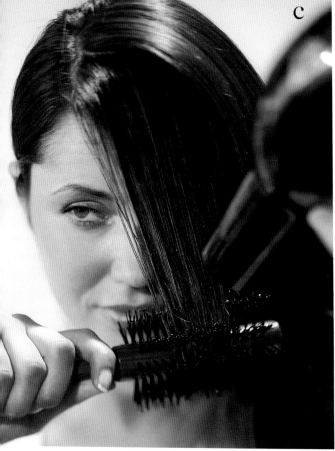

c

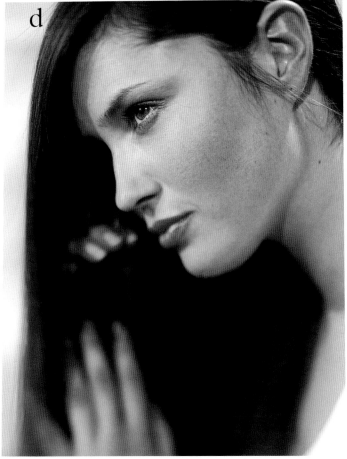

d

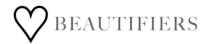

looking after your scalp

YOUR SCALP IS THE FIRST PLACE TO SHOW THE SIGNS OF STRESS WITHIN THE BODY. THAT'S BECAUSE DURING ILLNESS AND TIMES OF STRESS OR POOR NUTRITION, THE BODY COPES BY CONSERVING VITAL NUTRIENTS, AND THE FIRST PLACE IT STOPS SUPPLYING IS THE SCALP. NOT SURPRISINGLY, SCALP PROBLEMS CAN GO UNNOTICED OR IGNORED FOR SOME TIME. BUT ULTIMATELY A HEALTHY SCALP WILL PROMOTE HEALTHIER, THICKER HAIR, SO NOW'S THE TIME TO START TAKING NOTICE AND TREATING IT BETTER.

Wash hair more thoroughly
Washing regularly with a mild shampoo is vital. And ensure that you spend twice as long as you normally would on just rinsing it out. Many scalp problems are simply the result of a congested scalp so the clearer your scalp is the healthier it will be – and the healthier your hair as a result.

Improve your diet
Up your intake of oily fish and dark green vegetables. Cut down on white wine and dairy products, both renowned for aggravating conditions such as eczema, psoriasis and dandruff

Relax
Enjoy a scalp massage once or twice a week to help stimulate blood circulation to the scalp, especially if you've been under pressure or haven't been eating a well-balanced diet.

Acupuncture
Try it. It's proved very effective on stress-related, sensitive or itchy scalp conditions.

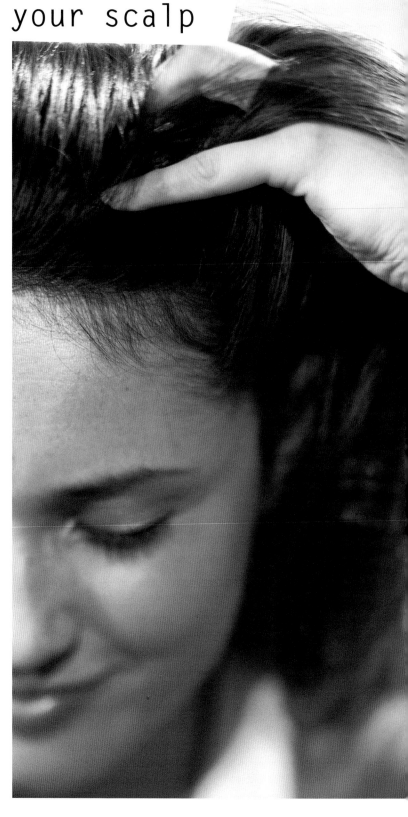

Soothing scalp massage

A RELAXING SCALP MASSAGE CAN INCREASE THE BLOOD FLOW TO NERVE ENDINGS TO BOOST THE SCALP. YOU CAN DO IT 'DRY' ANYTIME OR USING SCALP OIL IN STEP 4 FOR ADDED BENEFITS.

1 Sit in an upright, comfortable position, close your eyes and slowly relax your neck and shoulders (see page 75 or 224).

2 Use the tips of your index, middle and ring fingers together to massage gently, making tiny circles up both sides of your neck at once and along to the nape of your neck.

3 Working outwards from there, press both sets of fingers simultaneously along your hairline, until your fingers meet at the centre of your forehead.

4 Separate your fingers and place them all in your hair to massage the scalp gently.

5 Lift sections of your hair and pull ever so gently upwards, for a count of 3. Repeat several times.

Make your own stimulating, energizing and decongesting scalp oil (see page 220). Blend 10ml castor oil or grapeseed oil (the two finest water-soluble oils easily absorbed by the scalp) with a total of five drops of eucalyptus and/or rosemary essential oil. Dip your fingertips in the oil and use to massage into your scalp. Leave on for as long as possible and then rinse thoroughly.

Don't miss This feels even nicer if someone else does it to you.

conditioning hair mask

MUCH LIKE A FACE MASK, A HAIR MASK IS SIMPLY A MORE INTENSE CONDITIONER FOR YOUR HAIR. USE ONCE DURING YOUR 21-DAY PROGRAMME. IT TAKES ANYTHING FROM 5 TO 20 MINUTES TO ADD EXTRA SHINE AND BOOST CONDITION.

You can get deep-cleansing masks which contain mud to help remove any residue of hair styling products, moisturizing masks which help to replenish moisture and suppleness to dry ends, and protein masks which help to strengthen and 'rebuild' hair by conditioning the hair cuticle. Protein masks are perfect if your hair is dry from over-processing or too much sun as the proteins are absorbed under the cuticles and fill any gaps.

1 Apply to freshly washed, towel-dried hair that has had any excess water blotted out.

2 Leave on for the recommended time with a warm towel wrapped around your head. The extra warmth ensures that your hair absorbs as much product as possible, making it that much more effective. (Deep conditioning salon treatments always use warm lights to intensify the treatment.)

3 Rinse thoroughly and, if possible, allow your hair to dry naturally without using a hairdryer.

Protein masks For best results, apply before going into the bath (or steam room) as the heat will open up the cuticles and allow the ingredients to be absorbed more completely. And enhance the treatment by wrapping a sheet of cling film around your hair before the warm towel.

boosters

If you're going to have great-looking hair, treat these as essentials. Just once in this 21-day programme, a stylish, slightly 'edgy' cut and colour will take years off your face – and body – and help rediscover that more assertive, confident and vivacious new you.

colour your hair

WHETHER YOU WANT TO COVER UP LOTS OF GREY OR SUBTLY PERK UP YOUR NATURAL COLOUR AND ADD SHINE, NOTHING BEATS COLOUR. AND IT GIVES THAT EXTRA BOOST OF KNOWING THAT YOUR HAIR LOOKS GOOD.

Salon or home? Well, home's cheaper and quicker, but the finished effect is often a more solid block of colour rather than the intricate layering of two or three colours that a colourist would use to give a more natural effect. So if you want to add shine or subtly perk up your natural colour, do it at home. (Remembering that home colourants work best if you have medium to dark hair.) But the more colour you need – maybe you want to change your colour by two shades or more, or cover more than 50 per cent grey – then I'd recommend you go professional. A colourist can see all around your head (including the all-important back view), so your colour should be even as well as natural looking. She can also gauge which colour suits your skin tone so you have colour that's tailor-made to you.

If you're doing it yourself Unless you've decided on a complete colour change (in which case see a professional), keep within your own colour range for a natural effect. If in doubt, choose the next colour lighter or deeper than your own if it's your first attempt. When dyeing long or thick hair, buy a second kit to be sure you have enough.

● Product build-up can sometimes interfere with the colouring process, giving an uneven finish. Use a detoxifying shampoo beforehand for better results.
● Make sure you wear protective gloves.
● Do a strand test on some underneath hairs first. Dry hair is more porous – and that means it will soak up colour more rapidly – so you may need less time than the product specifies to achieve the colour you want.
● Use the colour mixture immediately. If the chemicals are left to oxidize before use, they may give a different result.

For the best, even coverage Work colour in well, from back to front, and separate your hair into 5cm (2in) sections as you go, rather than squeezing it all over and then trying to spread it. If your hair's longer than your chin, don't apply colour directly onto the ends – they're drier and more porous, and will absorb more colour than you'll want. Leave on for the desired amount of time, and then rinse thoroughly until water runs clear.

Which type do you need?

For subtle colour Choose a temporary, wash-in, wash-out colour (lasts 2–3 washes) that is best for brightening your own natural colour or semi-permanent (lasts between 8–10 washes). Semi-permanents temporarily coat your hair with a brighter version of your natural shade, and add some texture and body, and some condition too. They will turn grey into highlights.

For dramatic colour If you want something three shades or more away from your natural colour, then you need permanent or tone-on-tone colour. These work by lightening your natural hair colour first and then depositing a new colour on top.

Tone-on-tone colour (lasts up to 24 washes) is like semi-permanent except most contain a low level of hydrogen peroxide to lighten hair, making the colour last three times longer. They gradually fade with each wash, so 'tell-tale roots' aren't an issue.

Permanent colour (lasts until you cut it out) covers any amount of grey and lifts colour out of your hair, laying down a new shade. Roots are the problem so it's high maintenance. Highlights are permanent too, but they grow out subtly as they are random.

To look natural Keep within your own colour and skin tone range – red hair and olive skin won't fool anyone.

To cover grey Go for permanent colour but never darker than your own natural colour. Lighter shades are more flattering with age because your skin tone loses colour at the same time as your hair. Once you've gone grey, warm colour put back into your hair helps pale skin look healthier. So, if you were originally blonde, go golden (honey, gold and fawn shades); if you were originally brunette, go warmer (auburn, copper and chestnut shades).

Remember Preserve and protect new colour from sun, sea, chlorine, pollution and so on, and use haircare products specially formulated for coloured hair.

Why we go grey

Hair gets its colour from pigment produced by special cells (called melanocytes) in the hair follicles. With age these cells become less active so colour fades and our hair appears grey. Hair eventually turns white when these cells cease functioning altogether. A diet lacking in the essential hair vitamin B (depleted by stress) has also been found to accelerate grey. If in doubt, seek professional advice and bump up your intake of vitamin B.

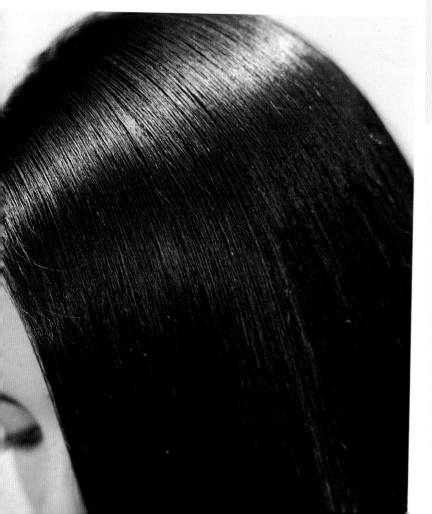

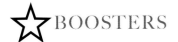

a great cut

A GREAT HAIRCUT CAN BE AS UPLIFTING AS COSMETIC SURGERY. IT MAY TAKE 21 DAYS TO DECIDE HOW YOU WANT YOUR HAIR TO LOOK, BUT IT'LL BE A MAXIMUM OF 3 HOURS (INCLUDING COLOUR) TO ACHIEVE IT. KEY FACTORS TO CONSIDER WHEN CHOOSING A NEW STYLE ARE ITS SUITABILITY TO YOUR HAIR TEXTURE, FACE SHAPE AND FEATURES, AND EASE OF MAINTENANCE. A HAIRSTYLIST CAN CUT AND BLOW-DRY A WOMAN'S HAIR TO MAKE IT LOOK FANTASTIC AS SHE LEAVES THE SALON, BUT IF SHE CAN'T MANAGE IT AT HOME, THERE'S NO POINT.

A classic bob is one of the most flattering styles for almost every hair type and face shape. And it can give the illusion of thicker hair for those who want to pump up the volume. You can vary its length, depending on how round or thin your face is. And if you have jowls, a longer length bob is more age-defying than cutting it shorter and showing them off. Only avoid a bob if you have very curly hair as it tends to lose the shape and can look old fashioned rather than stylish and modern.

A graduated bob is shaped around your face to soften the geometric look associated with a typical bob. Add a light fringe or feathering at the sides to soften features. For extra volume, graduate hair at the nape of the neck to lighten the load, coming forward to one length at the chin. If in doubt, start with a classic bob, and then work in some layers at your next appointment to vary the shape.

Long layers look very feminine and enable you to keep hair longer past 'a certain age'. Concentrate on hair condition by sticking to your new regular regime – with plenty of intensive conditioning treatments. The trick in styling is to 'shape' at the front rather than layer (which simply thins hair) so you avoid an unflattering 'curtain of hair' effect.

Short layers that frame the face suit most people, particularly those with petite features. It's gentler and more forgiving than severe scraped or slicked-back styles, and a halo of hair softens angular faces. Short layers also give the illusion of more body at the roots to lank or thinning hair.

Add a light fringe Nothing too heavy, just lightly feathered and soft – it will frame your face, looks quite young and flirty, and brilliantly hides frown lines. But avoid if your forehead is short.

And how to get it

Have a consultation Shop around recommended salons as you would for a new dress. Consultations should be free and you shouldn't feel obliged to anyone. Go when your hair looks most natural (i.e. you haven't just blow-dried curly locks straight against their will) and present yourself the way you want to look. Or a hairdresser will jump to the wrong conclusions about you and your tastes before you say a word.

Take photos This is especially important if you are trying out someone new. It will give both of you something to refer to in terms of shape, length and volume, and it also avoids miscommunication.

Be honest Say how much time you really spend on your hair. There's no point going for a look that takes an hour to perfect if you're only ever prepared to devote 5 minutes to your hair each day. And if you've had colour already, are on medication or are pregnant, say so. Your colour (even if it's your usual shade) may come out differently otherwise.

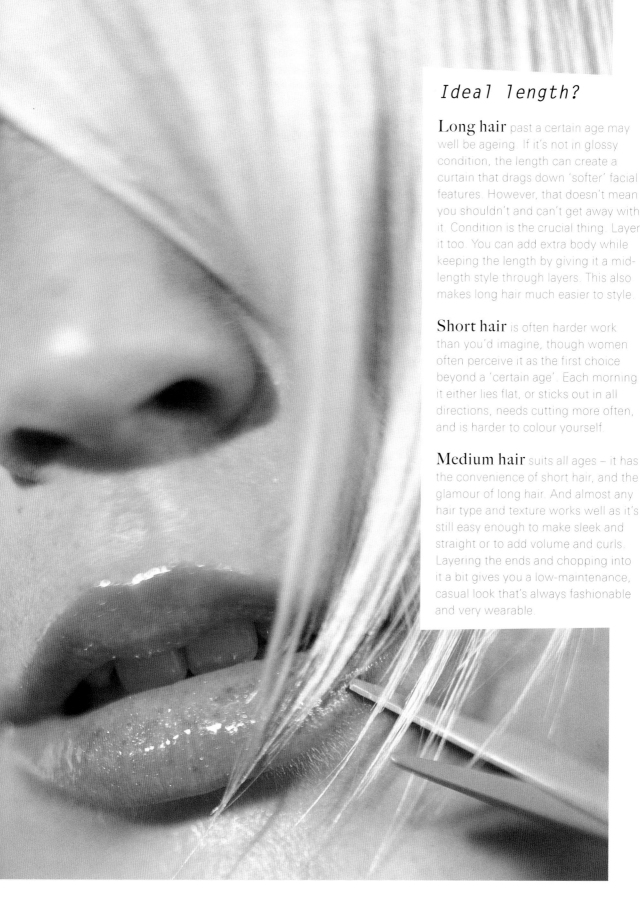

Ideal length?

Long hair past a certain age may well be ageing. If it's not in glossy condition, the length can create a curtain that drags down 'softer' facial features. However, that doesn't mean you shouldn't and can't get away with it. Condition is the crucial thing. Layer it too. You can add extra body while keeping the length by giving it a mid-length style through layers. This also makes long hair much easier to style.

Short hair is often harder work than you'd imagine, though women often perceive it as the first choice beyond a 'certain age'. Each morning it either lies flat, or sticks out in all directions, needs cutting more often, and is harder to colour yourself.

Medium hair suits all ages – it has the convenience of short hair, and the glamour of long hair. And almost any hair type and texture works well as it's still easy enough to make sleek and straight or to add volume and curls. Layering the ends and chopping into it a bit gives you a low-maintenance, casual look that's always fashionable and very wearable.

When your hair won't behave Spritz and damp down the outer layers, rather than shampoo the whole lot. You can then restyle in next to no time.

To curl the ends under When your hair is completely dry, spray a radial brush with light hairspray and use to roll the ends under. Heat with a dryer and hit the cooling button to lock in the curl before unrolling.

For smooth curls on dry hair Use dry heated rollers (the bigger the roller, the looser the curl). Brush your hair first, lightly spray with a setting lotion, comb through and then wind small sections of hair around each roller. Leave to cool totally, and then remove. Don't brush – just rub a tiny amount of serum between your fingers and smooth round each curl for more definition.

Flip the ends of your hair out Roll the hair around a radial brush and turn it under while blow-drying. Only at the end, when your hair's dry, do you reverse the roll and flip the curl out.

Velcro® rollers won't stay put? Pin them in place to stop them wobbling. If you allow them to fall out of place, you'll end up with a kink in your hair at the roots. To use Velcros to keep hair smooth, blow-dry hair first, and then distribute them throughout your hair.

To boost body any time Fluff hair with your fingers rather than a brush, which flattens. If your hair really needs brushing, do it from underneath with your head upside down. A couple of rollers on the crown can help boost volume at the roots, even when hair is very straight and flat.

fast track

To enhance your curls Use a diffuser attachment on your hairdryer. Choose a medium-heat setting – it's kinder to hair because it styles quickly as it dries, without being too hot. Overheating dehydrates your hair, making curls fluffy not curly.

Cut your hair regularly Aim for every six weeks (four if it's a short style). It keeps the sharpness of a cut (even if long), and reduces split ends. Regular cutting can also help to combat frizziness. Coarse grey hair benefits most from a short, sharp cut. Long frizzy hair needs more graduation, cutting hair away from the face to allow less frizzy hair to show from underneath.

Using straightening irons? Apply a leave-in conditioner on the ends after shampooing, blow-dry as straight as possible, and always use a medium setting on the irons to protect your hair from the intense heat.

Revive your hairstyle Tip your head upside down, spray the roots with a lightweight volumizing styling spray, allow 60 seconds to dry, and then throw back your head.

Revive your colour If your highlights tend to look brassy yellow, or your colour looks dull, it may be caused by metals in the water you wash it in. Brighten all-over colour and highlights using shampoo and conditioner for coloured hair.

How to refresh your hair When you need your hair to look good in a hurry, just wash the fringe and blow-dry: it takes 5 minutes. Make a centre parting and wash only the front triangle of hair (formed by the hairline with the apex at the parting) – this is the section that gets greasy and out of control first. And it's where other people's eyes are drawn when they look at you.

keeping it going

Choose a better path

There's no denying, remember, that your hair is forever on show – whether you're going out somewhere special or just popping down to the corner shop. And, as such, it immediately reflects the way you care not only for your hair, but for yourself. Much like hands and nails or feet, your hair reflects your love of yourself. It doesn't have to be long and glossy, just a regular cut to keep the shape, colour if it needs it, and the right products to help you shampoo and style on a daily basis.

Focus on the positive

It's how your hair makes you feel that counts. Soft, touchable hair that's in great condition is very sexy. And each part of you is just as important as any other – because feeling good about what you've achieved on the outside will add to all the positive changes you've achieved on the inside – it's that mind/body connection again.

Seek balance

Stay with the programme's main aim – to enhance your hair with a style that works with your hair – its texture, the way it really is – and see styling as a treat for special occasions. The less you 'do to it' in the salon, the stronger, healthier and easier to manage it will be. Chemical processes create great styles, but they're high maintenance, so until you really need colour, play with the one you have, using home wash-in wash-out vegetable dyes. Less maintainance on your part – more balance in your life.

Give yourself time

You'll have to get up 30–40 minutes earlier to shampoo and blow-dry your hair more frequently to keep that new you groomed and utterly gorgeous image. Sure, there'll be days you just tie it back for ease. But isn't it great knowing you can now make it look good any time you want?

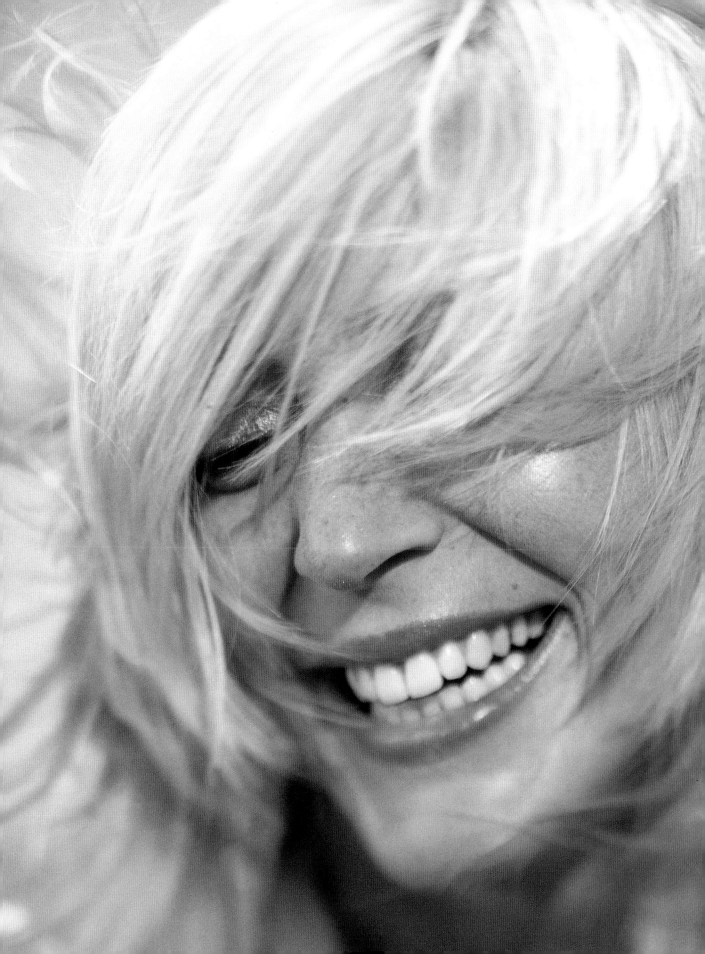

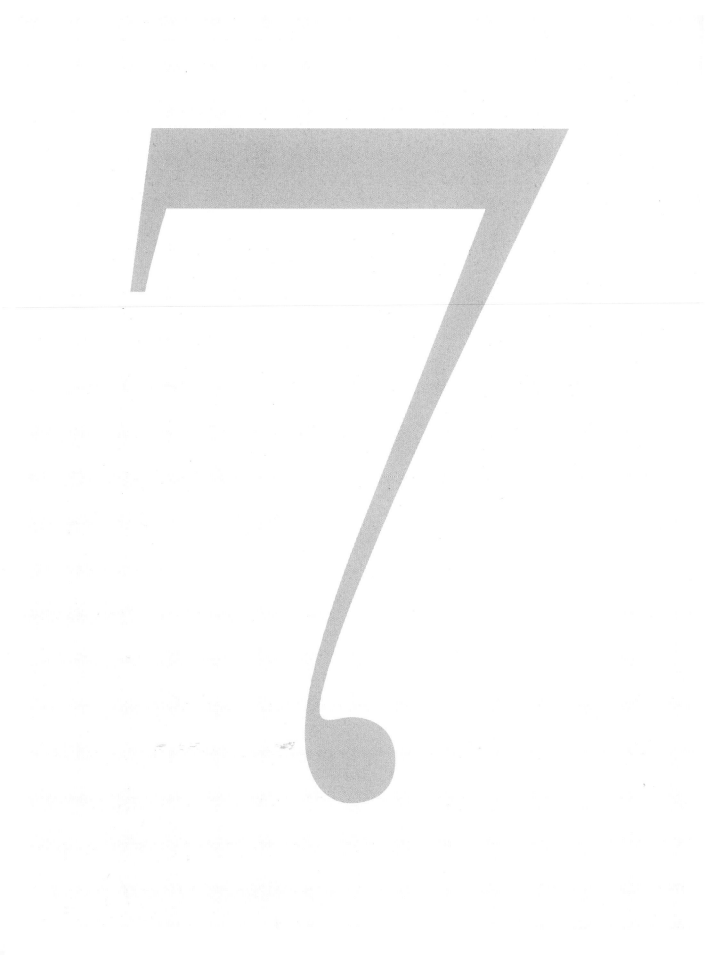

21 DAYS

TO

RELAXED

LIVING

Close your eyes. Breathe in deeply.
Imagine balance, happiness and peace
in every single aspect of your life.
That's a relaxed way of living.

Your
low-stress
programme

I guess this programme is all about learning to chill. Discovering how to relax so that you can deal with daily events and situations in a more serene state of mind. By building into your life a series of mind/body regimes and techniques designed to give you more self-control and self-belief, you learn to give everything you do more substance. So this programme is, above all, a way of revealing the new you by working from the inside out.

MIND OVER MATTER: IF YOU DON'T MIND, IT DOESN'T MATTER. APPLY THIS TO ALMOST EVERY ASPECT OF LIFE.

We're all doing too much
We work long and hard to improve our standard of living, but in the process are in danger of losing our capacity to enjoy life. A recent survey of work/life balance found that workers frequently sacrifice exercise, quality time with a partner, time with friends and social activities, and hobbies/entertainment to work longer hours. Yet these are all crucial aspects of life – known to promote mental health and to relieve mental-health problems when they do occur. We simply take too much upon ourselves. And the result is a whole horrendous catalogue of stress-related physical and psychological symptoms.

Remember
The way you think has a direct effect on how you look and feel. So seek a good state of mind.

Good stress and bad stress
Of course, these days 'stress' is a casual, throwaway term. And some stress is good for us. It's a part of excitement and anticipation; it's the power behind every creative thought and action. The time to take action in stressful situations is when the stress is not helping you to enjoy life.

Any of this sound familiar?
Early signs that stress is getting the better of you can range from headaches, neck and back pain, digestive disorders, constipation for some, diarrhoea in others, to irritable bowel syndrome (IBS), recurring colds and infections and heart palpitations. Others may develop habit changes (such as overeating and increased alcohol consumption, gambling and over-spending), coupled with mood swings through extreme anger, frustration and tears.

What you do in these 21 days

if you're 20-35...

You may be single or recently married, and if you have children they are probably quite small. Life is relatively straightforward, and your stress levels are mainly dependent on work life, finances and early relationship issues.

● Decide on a life plan. What do you want from life? What do you want to achieve?
● Organize – whether this means decluttering your home or sorting out financial papers, whatever would make life easier for you right now.
● Incorporate positive thinking – personal affirmations to remind yourself how important you are to you – and find techniques you feel comfortable with to combat stress and anxiety.
● Get good-quality sleep.
● Balance your blood-sugar levels (alcohol, chocolate, yo-yo eating habits are major culprits), using your Nutrition programme. And keep your spirits, energy and motivation up with all the other programmes.

...35-50

As we age, so do those around us. Be prepared for the loss of ageing parents. If you have children, you'll know that every aspect of their growing up is stressful to some extent. And child-rearing years place heavy demands on your relationship so you may experience problems here. If you work, you will either be established in what you do or seeking a new career. Change is good – but stressful.

● Learn to enjoy your children more. Play with them more – it's what they want, too. Children are great stress-busters as well as stress-builders.
● Practise positive thinking. A calm, contented parent builds a stronger, relaxed child.
● Seek order in every aspect of your life. Use the de-stressing strategies (see pages 218–19).
● Try something new – relaxation classes maybe or a mind/body fitness technique.

...50 and over

Loss of loved ones is even more likely now, and bereavement is a major cause of stress. Work may be stressful too, with redundancy or retirement on the horizon.

● Have the children left home? Get a pet, renowned for reducing stress in humans!
● Make time for your friends and family. Have no regrets about telling those you love how you feel. This makes bereavement, when it comes, easier to handle.
● Think positively. Make more of each day. Start the day fresh, and focus on winding down at the end of the day.
● Maintain regular exercise at a moderate pace and a nourishing, healthy eating plan to boost your Low-stress programme.

What you'll achieve

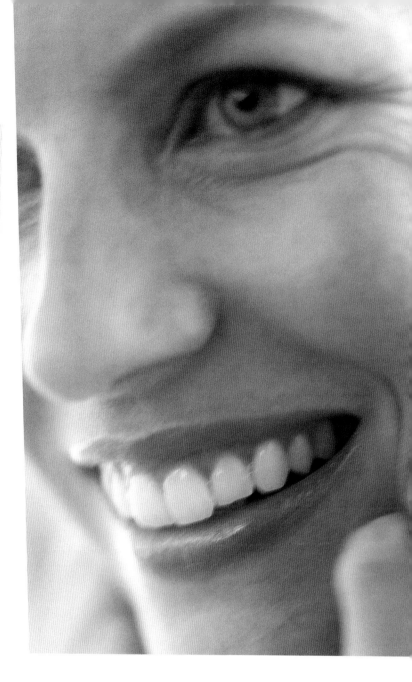

A positive attitude The Low-stress programme, like everything else in this book, is taking you towards one ultimate goal – to be contented, happy and living your life to the max. A positive, happy nature is good for you and for others. Research shows that laughter releases your body's pain relief – endorphins and enkephalins – to speed up its own healing processes. Indeed, laughter has even been referred to as 'internal massage' because it is proven to exercise the heart, lungs and central nervous system. And, in much the same way as someone who feels down can bring us down too, being around happiness makes us all feel happier.

Less 'bad' stress You'll learn how to help yourself gain control over the causes and effects of bad stress on your mind and body without having to resort to constant cups of coffee and a high sugar intake. Using the de-stressing and calming techniques in this Low-stress programme, supported by your Nutrition and Fitness programmes, you'll be better equipped to deal with the times when stress is really not helping you, and you feel overwhelmed by it.

More balance in your life Knowing how to calm and focus your mind on mental and physical relaxation will bring significant rewards in many aspects of your life.
● Armed with a greater capacity for self-control, you'll be free to follow your ambitions and achieve so much more.
● By learning to focus on your positives and seeking less perfection in yourself, you really will reduce destructive self-criticism. And that's then reflected in the way others perceive you and relate to you.
● In writing everything down – how you feel, areas in your life you're happy with, and areas that you're not – you help create clarity and that can make you all the more realistic about problems and solutions.

your low-stress kit

Camomile tea

Or other herbal teas, such as fennel, nettle and dandelion. These can subtly lift or calm your mood as well as being extremely cleansing for your body during the Nutrition programme. However, do be cautious with any herbal tea if you are on medication as they are highly stimulating.

Essential oils

Lavender, geranium, peppermint, rosemary, rose and camomile are the key mood-enhancing essential oils for relaxation (see page 220). And you'll already be using energizing and relaxing essential oils in your Bodycare programme (see page 124). Vetiver, another of the relaxers, is also known to relieve depression and promote better sleep. It's vital that you like the aroma of the oil you use, because the more positively it affects your mind, the better your mood. Go to a health-food shop to experience a few of the aromas. Waft samplers well away from your nose, and bear in mind that, although these oils smell strong, their scent is softer once they are blended with carrier oil or water.

Candles

Use them to create an atmosphere of relaxation. Arranging candles of different heights creates a heavenly ambience. If you like scented candles, choose ones that either match your favourite perfume or have a subtle aromatherapy scent. There's nothing worse than polluting your tranquil scene with an aroma you can't bear. Right now, harmony is everything.

Notebook

Keep it with you throughout the day to record 'positive' thoughts on how you're doing, what you've enjoyed, what you'll never try again. Keep your daily planner taped in the back each week for ease. Add photocopies of useful mini rituals, such as your deep-breathing ritual, time-managing tips, and techniques to up your energy and brain power.

A peaceful space

Above all things, you need to find yourself a place that you can return to again and again and that you associate with the sensations of calm and tranquillity. It may be a particular room in your home or a corner in a room (just as Buddhists use temple areas to meditate and contemplate peace), even a particular chair. Or perhaps a space outside the home. Here you must be able to withdraw for small moments of time – away from partners and family – to be silent and peaceful, just like the space itself.

Vaporizer

Choose between an electric vaporizer, which blows air through the oil, or an oil burner, which heats up the oil, using a candle. Either will help to fill the air around you with the essential oil of your choice – you can mix a couple too, providing they have the same properties (that is, both are relaxant or stimulant), though lavender mixes well with all oils. Diffusing oils is especially effective if you are particularly sensitive to essential oils. Check the health-precaution advice on page 220.

transformers

To adopt a more harmonious lifestyle, you need to create peaceful spaces throughout the day to reflect. They're just moments in time, but time that you might otherwise spend feeling harassed. Each and every new day you need to seek out ways to stop the clock and unwind.

wake-up moments

THESE LITTLE GESTURES CAN AFFECT THE MOOD YOU'RE IN FROM THE WORD GO. TRY TO INCORPORATE A FEW OF THEM INTO EACH NEW DAY. IT'S A WAY OF SHOWING YOURSELF THAT YOU'RE REALLY GOING TO GIVE YOUR NEW YOU PROGRAMME ALL YOUR BEST.

● Put your bedroom light on a timer to turn on an hour before you wake. According to psychologists, the small amount of light that enters the retina before you wake inhibits the release of melatonin (the biorhythm hormone that makes you tired and sleepy), so you eventually wake up brighter, more energetic and in a better mood.

● Wake up to music. Music can make our spirits light but, even more significantly, singing along re-activates the creative side of your brain (the right side) so you'll feel more energized for the day. Just make sure it's selected music and not simply the distracting noise of a radio station constantly interrupted by adverts.

● As soon as you do wake, pull back the curtains and enjoy the light. As more daylight enters the retinas of your eyes, further inhibiting the release of melatonin, so your mood and energy levels should begin to soar.

● Appeal to your senses. Diffuse lemon, grapefruit or mandarin essential oil in a vaporizer in your bedroom to perk you up. Spritz your sheets with a lemon-water spray (eight drops of lemon oil in 50ml water). And don't forget to use those citrus scents later in the shower (see page 123).

● Remember your morning detoxifying mug of hot water and lemon or herbal tea (see chapter 1). Carry it back to your bedroom and take regular little sips as you perform your daily skincare regime. I like rubbing my teeth with the lemon peel afterwards, to whiten them. But brush your teeth quickly to reduce any acidity on the enamel.

Time for you Silence is golden... and very rare (especially with a young family around). If you find it hard to lock yourself away for quiet moments to practise your breathing rituals and other relaxing therapeutic treats, arrange half-hour time slots with your partner, or choose a time when the children have gone to bed.

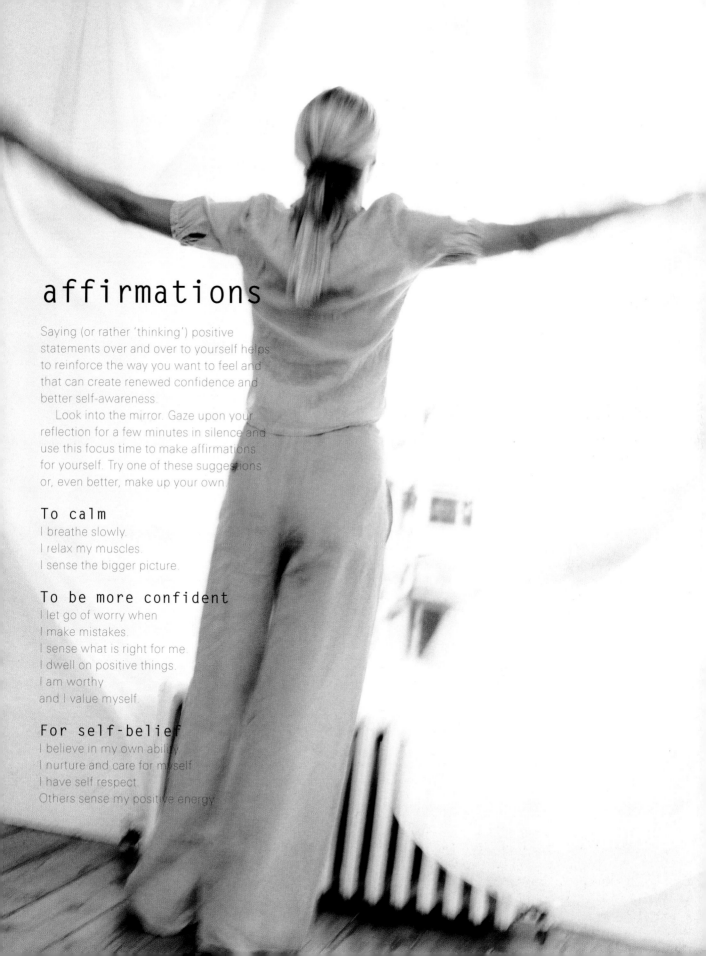

affirmations

Saying (or rather 'thinking') positive
statements over and over to yourself helps
to reinforce the way you want to feel and
that can create renewed confidence and
better self-awareness.

Look into the mirror. Gaze upon your
reflection for a few minutes in silence and
use this focus time to make affirmations
for yourself. Try one of these suggestions
or, even better, make up your own.

To calm

I breathe slowly.
I relax my muscles.
I sense the bigger picture.

To be more confident

I let go of worry when
I make mistakes.
I sense what is right for me.
I dwell on positive things.
I am worthy
and I value myself.

For self-belief

I believe in my own ability.
I nurture and care for myself.
I have self respect.
Others sense my positive energy.

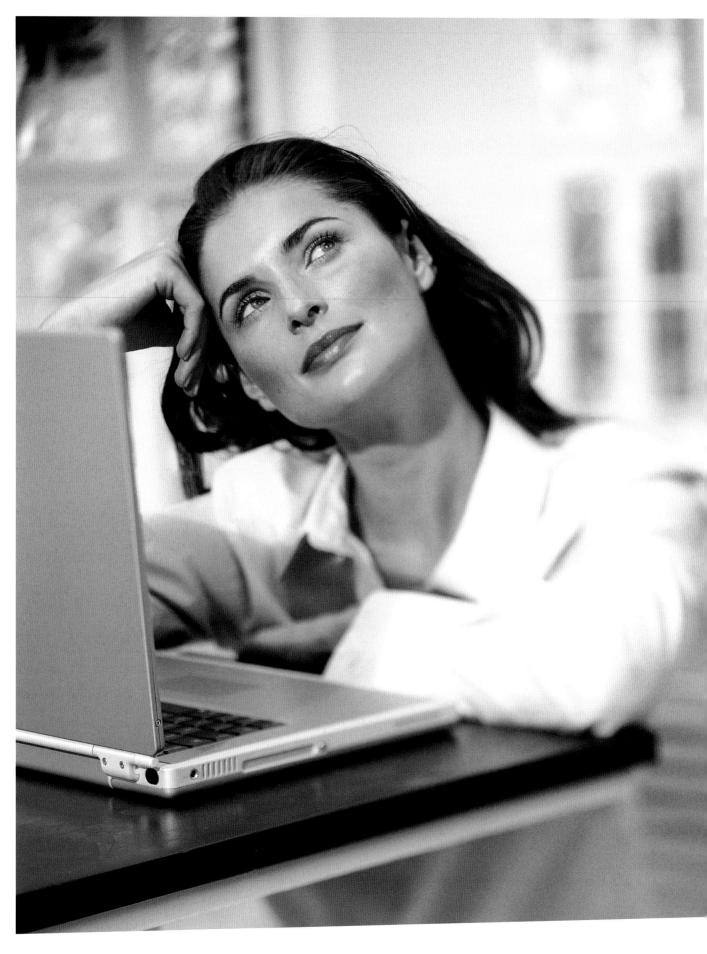

midday moments

Losing concentration at your desk? No patience with the children? Create a quiet moment to reflect, think and breathe with these mind/body techniques.

Relax your body Tension can grip your body any time of day. Without realizing, you may grit your teeth for control in times of anger, clench the steering wheel, hunch your shoulders and screw up your eyes in deep concentration. But simply relax your muscles, and you de-stress your mind, body and spirit in one.

Take a break Deep breathing is the best way to calm your body when you are under pressure. Try this exercise. Sit upright in a comfortable chair, with your hands resting on your stomach. Breathe in fully, count to 2, and then breathe out for a count of 6 at the same rate. Be aware of your hands rising and falling. Repeat twelve times.

Take a walk Get some air and walk off the way you feel – there, in 20 minutes you've already done a workout.

Think positive You are what you believe. In the same way that you are what you eat, so you are what you think. And you can only believe what you tell yourself. Practise those affirmations (see page 209), and learn to celebrate every aspect of your life.

Just be Often when you feel overloaded by every aspect of your life, you need to just take a step back from the daily routine and simply switch off. A positive outlook frees the mind, body and spirit, but it is often only by letting go that you can see beyond the obstacles placed before you. Now is the time to let go. Make space to allow the joy of living back into your life each and every day and you will feel renewed and energized once more. To be spirited, you need spirit.

Try mind mapping Improve your memory, creativity and concentration by stimulating your brain with a litttle 'mind mapping'. On a piece of paper, practise organizing information you want to remember in order of importance or hierarchy – just like a family tree. Ask youself the basic seven questions any journalist uses when covering a story: what, who, when, why, where, how and which? And you'll be amazed by how clear and organized everything soon becomes.

An hour for lunch

Squeeze in a therapeutic mind/body treatment at least once in your 21-day programme. Find a therapist near your office or home.

Aromatherapy massage uses fragrant essential oils from a wide variety of flowers, plants and herbs to relax, revitalize or rebalance the whole being.

Acupuncture uses needles inserted in very specific energy points throughout the body in order to stimulate its own healing mechanisms.

Reflexology is the diagnostic massage technique used to stimulate specific energy points on the soles of the feet, thereby helping to restore energy flow throughout the body.

Reiki is a healing therapy using relaxation and spiritual energy to restore calm and balance.

Shiatsu is a form of massage that uses fingertip pressure along energy channels (or meridians) that, it is believed, run on the surface of the body but also connect at deeper levels with the functions of different organs.

wind-down moments

How often do you take time to reflect on the positive events of the day? Most of us rarely stop to consider the daily marvels - beauty in nature, the innocence and laughter of a child, the kindness of others, even achievement through our own efforts. Take time each evening to wind down.

Wipe away tension from your brows with a quick but very effective massage. Dabble the tips of your middle fingers in a calming mix of two drops each of rose and lavender essential oil in 10ml (1 tbsp) almond carrier oil. After inhaling the aroma for a few moments, place your fingertips on the inner ends of your eyebrows. Gently but firmly with small, upward movements, brush along the length of your brows. Then, starting again from the inner ends, press your fingertips firmly at several points along the browline. Brush again. Inhale the aroma once more and relax.

Enjoy a cup of camomile tea to relax the body and ease digestion at the end of the day.

Spritz a little of your favourite fragrance on your sheets. Or make up your own sleepy aromatherapy spray: a total of eight drops of vetiver, lavender and geranium in 50ml water.

Avoid watching TV in bed, especially over these three weeks. It can be over-stimulating to your mind when really you need to focus on relaxing.

Focus on everything you're doing right Use those precious moments before sleep comes to consider how much you have achieved in the day and what extra treatment you can fit in to make tomorrow even better. Keep a record in your notebook so you can compare your thoughts each evening.

Fit in more quality sleep

Make 11pm your curfew. Although individual sleep needs vary, between six and a half and eight hours a night is the norm.

We are all living lives with increasing pressures, and it's easy to perceive sleep as being less important than it is. But a recent Australian study showed that a single sleepless night has just the same effect on co-ordination, judgement and reaction time (especially important if you are driving) the following day as the consumption of the recommended weekly alcohol limit (21 units for men, 14 for women) in one sitting. And recent Canadian research has also indicated that for every two hours of sleep below a standard eight your IQ is lowered by two points per night. So people who skimp on sleep every night for a week – sleeping, say, just six hours each night – may feel reasonably OK, but their IQs will have decreased by no less than 14 points at the end day 7.

The good news is that if you do need to skimp on your sleep experts say a siesta-like 'power nap' of 15 or 20 minutes during the day can reboot your mental alertness for quite a few hours. Just think how those holiday afternoon snoozes restore body and soul. So put yourself in holiday mode. And even if you're not low on sleep, book in for the occasional afternoon nap if you can.

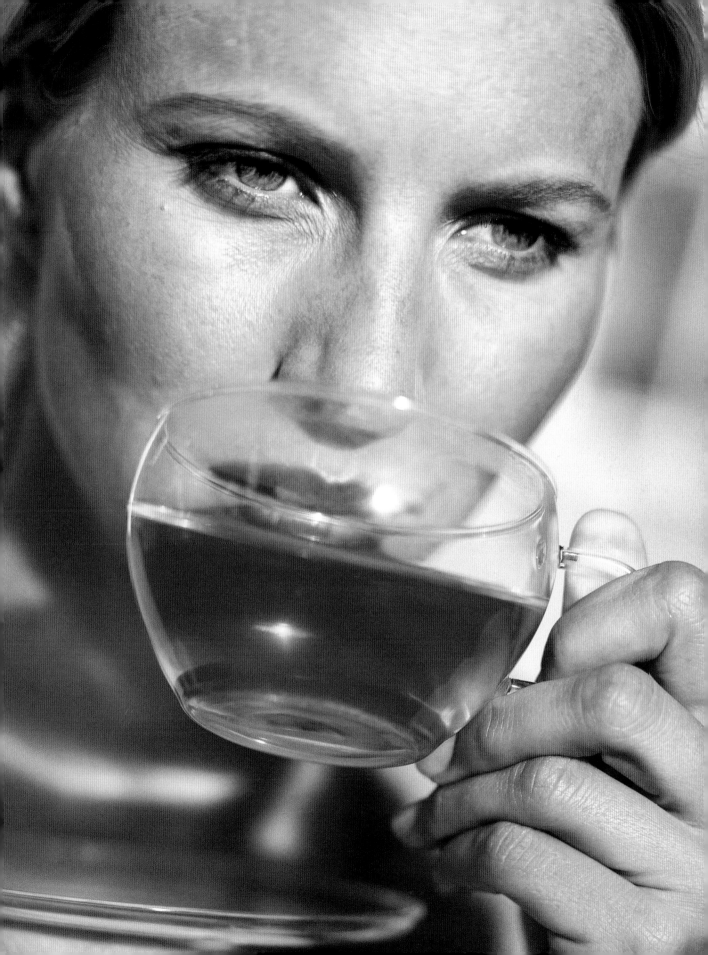

boosters

Anything that helps to create calm, peace and order in your life will boost your energy, vitality and mood, and plays a vital part in this programme. Use these skills to banish chaos in your head and heart, and focus your mind on the positive at all times, even when times seem hard.

your breathing ritual

TIME TO LEARN HOW TO BREATHE DEEPLY AND RHYTHMICALLY. ONCE YOU'VE MASTERED THE TECHNIQUE YOU CAN 'BREATHE' ANYWHERE, ANYTIME – IT NEED ONLY TAKE 5-10 MINUTES – THOUGH IT'S ESPECIALLY EFFECTIVE IN A PEACEFUL ENVIRONMENT, AND IN BED.

We were born to do it so you'd think by now we'd know how to breathe properly. But many of us are using less than half our total lung capacity when we breathe. And when we're stressed we resort to shallow breathing, which is totally the opposite of how we should breathe, and only makes us more anxious. Still need convincing? Well, you'll find that people who practise breathing principles such as yoga, t'ai chi or pilates are more focused and calm in their approach to life.

1 Lie on your back on the floor, with your legs slightly apart, toes facing outward, and your arms a little away from your sides, palms upwards. (You may want to use a yoga mat for comfort.)

2 Concentrate for a minute on relaxing all your limbs. Feel your backbone lengthen.

3 Take a deep breath in through your nose while keeping your body without tension: your abdomen should rise and expand as you fill with air. Breathe out through your mouth and your tummy falls.

4 Rest both your hands very lightly on your lower abdomen, palms downward. Focus simply on their rise and fall in tune with your breathing as you breathe in and out ten times.

5 In this position, imagine the air you breathe is a sparkling white light and with each inward breath it travels all round your body. You're filling your whole self with oxygen. Hold that sense of the air within your body for each breath and then slowly let it go, following its journey from the base of your abdomen up to your mouth.

6 Move your hands up to the base of your ribs. Keep your shoulders and arms relaxed and feel the open stretch right across your ribs as you breathe deeply and slowly in and out ten times, all the time sensing your breath through your fingertips.

7 Place both hands on your chestbone. And again breathe in and out deeply, feeling in pace and at peace with your precious breath. After all, it gives you life – what could be more vital to you?

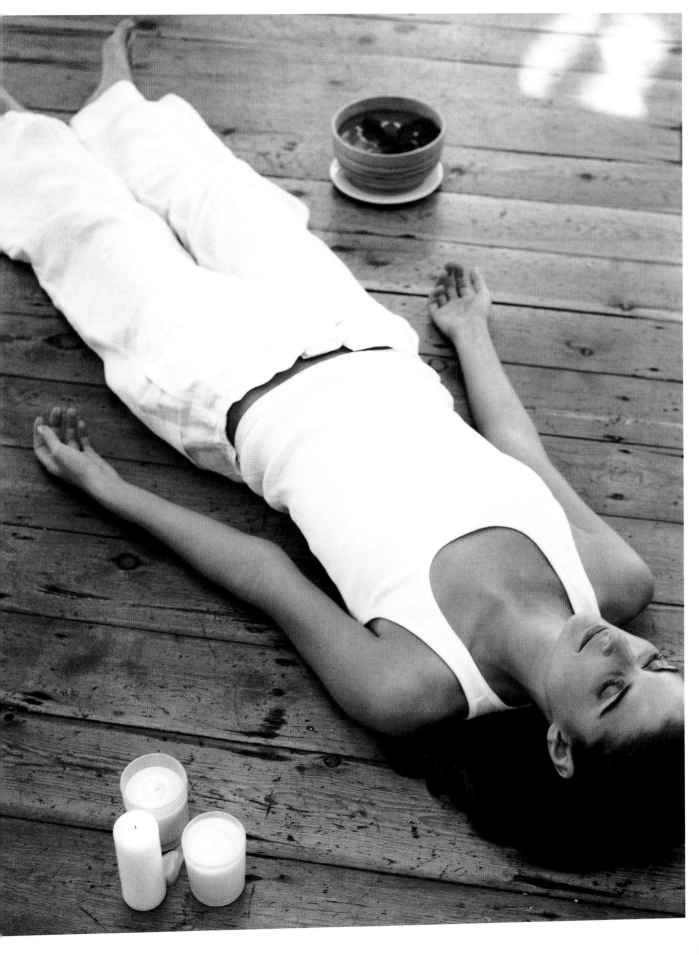

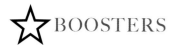
your morning feel-good stretch

IF YOU'RE GOING TO START THE DAY AFRESH, THIS CLASSIC MORNING YOGA RITUAL, CALLED THE SUN SALUTATION, IS A MUST. DO IT BEFORE YOUR EARLY-MORNING STRETCH (SEE CHAPTER 2). IT STIMULATES ENERGY FLOW AS IT STRETCHES EVERY SINGLE MUSCLE GROUP IN YOUR BODY – A PERFECT WAY TO SET YOU UP FOR THE DAY.

Practise until the sequence flows from step to step, action to action, as one unified movement. The breathing pattern is important too: it's in and out through your nose, breathing in as you begin a new part of the sequence and then breathing out with each stretch. I've suggested a count of 3 for each hold, but work at your own pace, holding for less if it helps.

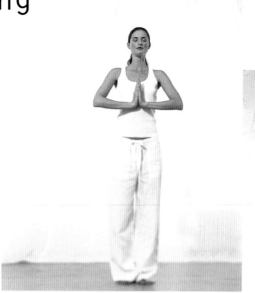

a

b

1   Stand, shoulders relaxed, back straight, tummy in, feet together and your hands in front of you at chest level, palms together as in a prayer position (as shown, a). Take four or five deep breaths in and out before beginning the sequence.

2   Breathe in, and then breathe out as you stretch your arms, palms still together, above your head (as shown, b). Hold for a count of 3.

3   Breathe in, and out as you bend forwards from the hips, reaching down toward the floor to hold your ankles (as shown, c) and bringing your head as close to your legs as is comfortable. Hold for a count of 3.

4   Breathe in, and out as you place your hands on the floor in front of you and then stretch your left leg backwards, toes turned under, while you bend your right knee to form a right angle (as shown, d). Hold for a count of 3. (Don't over-stretch yourself: keep your left leg slightly bent at the knee if you aren't quite flexible enough – you soon will be.)

5 Breathe in, and out as you extend your right leg back too, feet hip-width apart, while you flex your spine downward and lift your chest and head upward away from the floor. Hold for a count of 3. Try to stay on your toes if you can.

6 Breathe in, and out as you bring your head down between your arms and push your bottom into the air to create an inverted 'V' with your body (as shown, e). Hold for a count of 3.

7 Breathe in, and out as you swiftly raise your head up again and bring your left leg up to place the foot on the floor between your hands, with your knee forming a right angle, just as you did in step 4. Hold for a count of 3.

8 Breathe in, and out as you reverse the whole sequence of movements and holds – first your right leg back up, then your hands by your ankles, followed by standing tall with your arms above your head, and finally back to the prayer position.

c

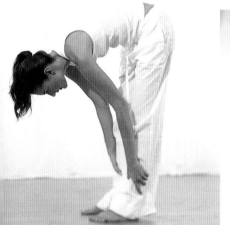

d

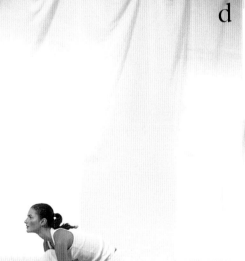

e

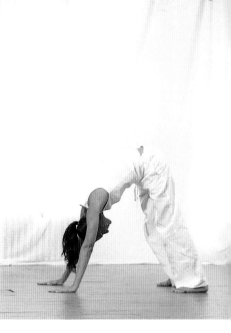

manage your time

ONE OF THE BIGGEST STRESSES OF MODERN LIFE IS THAT WE NOW HAVE
SO MANY OPTIONS OPEN TO US THAT WE JUST DON'T KNOW HOW TO FIT
EVERYTHING IN. BUT LEARN HOW TO USE TIME MORE EFFECTIVELY - BY
RE-ASSESSING YOUR HABITS, MAKING A FEW POSITIVE ADJUSTMENTS -
AND YOU HAVE A GREAT DE-STRESSING STRATEGY AT YOUR FINGERTIPS.

● Make a list of weekly home and work tasks and allocate each one to a
regular time-slot. Never depart from this unless absolutely necessary, and
do not allow anyone else to change your routine for you.

● Make a note of extra tasks when they are requested or required. A poor
memory can be responsible for doing the same thing twice – a total waste
of time – and for creating disorder.

● Learn how to say 'no'. How many times do you accept invitations to go
somewhere out of politeness and end up resenting the wasted time?
Don't act out of obligation – do things because YOU want to do them, not
to please others.

● If you have a large task, split it up into several smaller tasks. And tick
each one off as you complete it. This way you'll feel a sense of progress
rather than being overwhelmed by the enormity of what you have to do.

● Delegate and don't look back. It's pointless passing some task – at work
or at home – on to someone else if you're then going to interfere with its
progress. Walk away until it's done.

● Set yourself realistic time limits. There's nothing like a deadline to make
you perform more effectively.

● Prioritize. There is only so much that you can accomplish in a day.
Make a daily list of 'stuff-to-do' – those needed by midday at the top.

● Don't strive for perfection, accept your limitations, and recognize what
you've achieved each day.

Avoid procrastination.
Don't put anything off. Do
the tough job at its allotted
time – tomorrow may be
even busier. Your new
regime is to tackle it now.

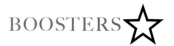

create order

TIME TO SIMPLIFY YOUR LIFE. THIS MEANS FOCUSING ON THE IMPORTANT THINGS, AND GETTING RID OF ANYTHING THAT MERELY TAKES UP TIME, SPACE, MONEY OR ENERGY. GET RID OF THE OBSTACLES THAT ARE STOPPING YOU FROM REACHING YOUR GOALS. ADOPT A 'CAN DO' ATTITUDE TO LIFE.

How much time do you waste each week looking for things that you can't find because you have so much 'stuff'? If you're looking for extra time, get rid of all your excess stuff and see how much time you save.

● Spend just a few minutes EVERY day organizing and tidying up. Have a place for everything. Make the effort to put things in their place as soon as you finish with them.

● Set aside some time each week to file all your paperwork. A small amount of time spent each week saves a big panic when it comes round to filling in your tax return.

● Stop generating clutter! Start using the 'one-in-one-out' rule. Every time you bring something into the house, take the equivalent out. So, each time you buy five magazines, get rid of five from last month so clutter never gets a chance to build up. If you want to go a step further, start using the 'one-plus-one-more' rule. Same as above, but if you buy two new books, three have to go! Wherever you can, try to recycle or give suitable items to charity.

● Do Direct Debit. This means you'll feel more in control of your finances. You'll never have to remember to pay bills on time and it saves you all those time-wasting trips to the post box or bank, together with the cost of stamps and envelopes.

● Don't spend what you haven't got. Do an accurate account of your expenditure each month. If you have been worrying about finances, this is the best way to work out how you are spending your money, ways to cut back on non-essentials, and whether you need to downsize.

Don't miss When you create space, there is more room for good things to come into your life.

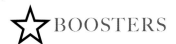

aromatherapy

EVEN IF YOU THINK YOU HAVE NEVER COME ACROSS ESSENTIAL OILS BEFORE, YOU WILL HAVE EXPERIENCED AROMATHERAPY. EVERY TIME YOU PEEL AN ORANGE OR SLICE A LEMON, THE ZESTY ESSENTIAL OIL IS RELEASED, MAKING YOU FEEL A LITTLE MORE ALERT AND ALIVE.

Aromatherapy is the mind/body treatment that uses pure essential oils, extracted from plant material – flowers, fruits and the bark or resin of many trees. It can restore emotional balance and help combat anxiety and insomnia, as well as healing many common ailments, and in particular skin infections, hormonal imbalance and everyday muscular aches and pains.

Essential oils are composed of very complex chemicals with the power to affect that part of the brain known as the lymbic system (which controls memories and emotions). They can be absorbed through the skin directly into the bloodstream or inhaled. Either way you can enhance your mood in next to no time.

The easiest and most beneficial ways to use essential oils are in the bath, as a massage oil or by using an electric vaporizer or oil burner. But, because these oils are so potent, most need to be diluted (either in water or in a 'carrier' oil) if they are to come in contact with the skin. See Don't miss (below) for exceptions.

Bath Use six to ten drops of pure essential oil, or one to two capfuls of a blend (that is, one or more essential oils mixed in a carrier oil such as almond, wheatgerm or grapeseed oil). Add to the bath once the water has run, and step in immediately.

Massage Add a total of five drops of your chosen essential oil to every 10ml (1tbsp) of carrier oil. Rub between your hands, inhale and then massage into your skin to relax or rejuvenate.

Vaporizer Follow the instructions for the type you choose (see page 206) Or improvise, adding a few drops of esssential oil to a bowl of warm water.

Inhalation Dot one or two drops of your chosen essential oil onto a tissue, and inhale at frequent intervals. Or follow the instructions for steaming in the Skincare programme (see page 98).

Stock up on the essentials

Camomile calms the body and soothes the soul. Drink it (as a tea), bathe in it (blended with lavender and geranium – two drops of each), inhale it.

Geranium, an effective sedative, relieves both anxiety and fatigue.

Lavender rebalances – either by relaxing or lifting your mood.

Peppermint clears and refreshes the brain and increases mental alertness.

Rose is emotionally uplifting, helping to boost confidence, beat stress and relieve tension. (It's also fab for dry, mature skins.)

Rosemary helps you to focus or to stay awake against all odds when situations demand it.

Don't skimp Check the label says 'pure essential oil'. If it also gives the plant derivative (the botanical name in Latin), the company probably takes time to source the plant species, thereby providing good-quality oil. And there's another way to check too: pure essential oils do not leave oily marks! Put a drop on a piece of paper – if there's an oily mark after a short while, the oil has been diluted with vegetable oil so it will not be as effective.

Don't miss Because of their potency, essential oils should always be used in the correct concentration. And they should never be applied to the skin neat – the only exceptions are lavender and tea tree. If you are pregnant or suffer from asthma, high blood pressure or epilepsy, always consult a qualified practitioner before using any essential oil. Keep essential oils well out of the reach of children.

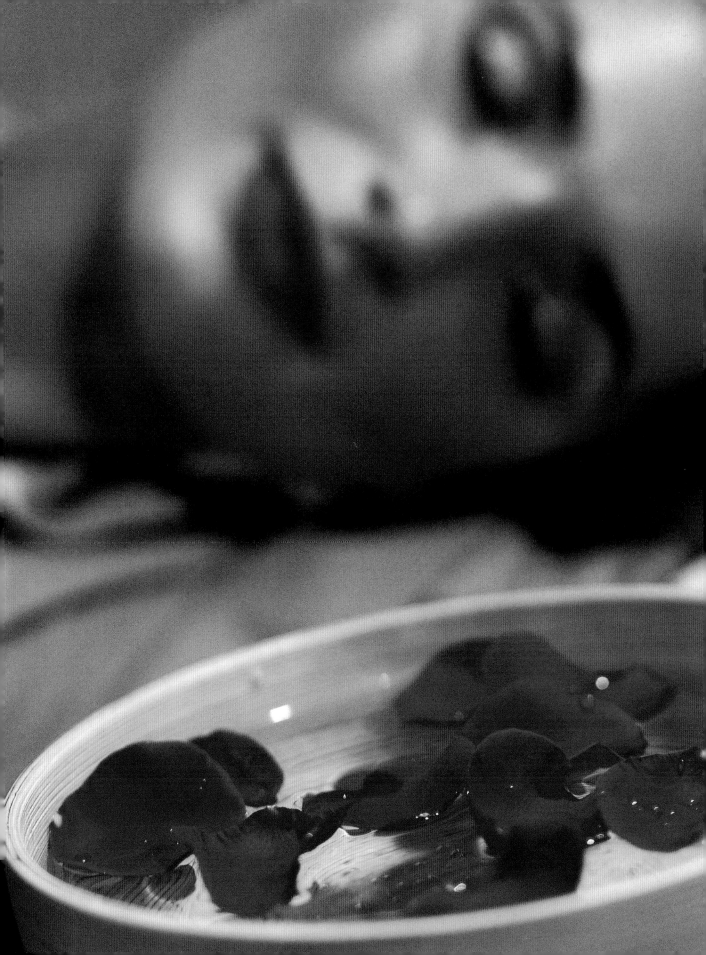

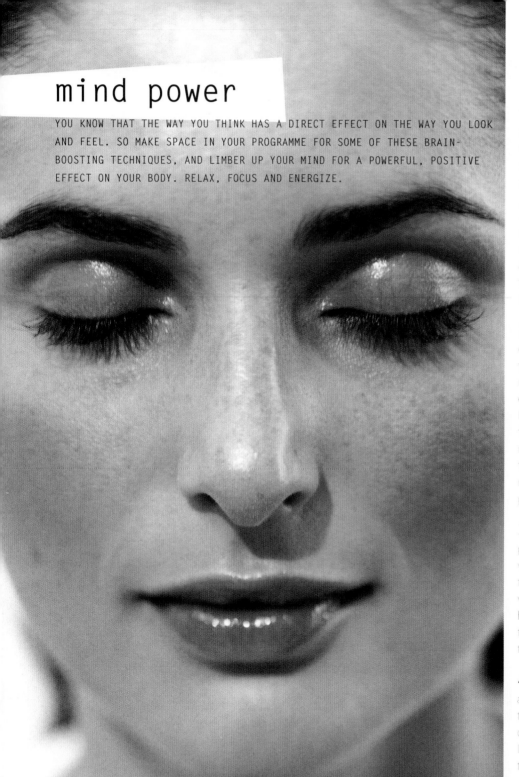

mind power

YOU KNOW THAT THE WAY YOU THINK HAS A DIRECT EFFECT ON THE WAY YOU LOOK AND FEEL. SO MAKE SPACE IN YOUR PROGRAMME FOR SOME OF THESE BRAIN-BOOSTING TECHNIQUES, AND LIMBER UP YOUR MIND FOR A POWERFUL, POSITIVE EFFECT ON YOUR BODY. RELAX, FOCUS AND ENERGIZE.

Visualize

The art of relaxation through mental imagery will enhance the breathing ritual (see page 214) once you get the hang of it

1 Find a comfortable position. This may be lying propped up on cushions in a candlelit room, sitting in your favourite armchair or lying back in a warm bath.

2 Once you are breathing deeply and regularly, close your eyes and focus your mind on a beautiful, happy or peaceful place. This can be anywhere that is special for you – on a beach, in a rainforest or on a hill top in the Lake District (that's mine) – anywhere that's positive for you.

3 Create a mental picture of the way it was when you were last there – the warmth of the sun on your skin, the scenery, the happiness you felt – and then imagine yourself there once again

4 Keep your breath deep and regular and stay like this for as long as you are comfortable – but no longer than 20 minutes in the bath.

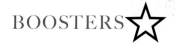

Meditate

This is the ultimate mind, body and soul therapy. Once you've learned 'how to', you will find it's the best antidote to stress. Research consistently shows that meditation can slow down the heart rate and breathing, lower blood pressure, boost your immune system and reduce muscle tension and headaches – all of which are stress-related. And it also clears the mind and gives you new focus and power – mind power – from within. Here's one method. Try it for 15–20 minutes a day.

1 Choose somewhere quiet, sticking to the same place at first will help to concentrate your mind on your intent.

2 Adopt a comfortable position, Lie, for example, on your back, your hands by your sides, palms facing upward; seated makes it less likely you will fall sleep. Choose an object to hold if it helps you focus more easily. This can be anything – a smooth pebble, a crystal (rose quartz is a therapeutic stone), a locket.

3 Rely on something simple to mark the beginning and end of each session. A hum, a word spoken, a bell, a huge sigh, whatever. Avoid music.

4 Close your eyes and breathe deeply for a few minutes. Now imagine a white light entering your body through the very top of your head. With your eyes still closed, try to 'see' the colour white and let it fill your head , which slowly in turn feels almost weightless. Concentrate on letting this light flood down your spine and filter out into your arms and legs, fingertips and toes.

5 Once your body is flooded with white light, focus on allowing it to travel back the way it came. Pause at several points as it moves up the centre of your body, letting the light form a colour – any colour – each time it rests.

6 Continue until the white light reaches the top of your head and then slowly release it into the space beyond. When it has finally gone, rest for just a moment before gradually opening your eyes.

Stimulate

You've no doubt heard the phrase 'Use it or lose it'? Use your brain – keeping it busy and active well into old age – and you will almost certainly feel and act younger for much longer. Cease to be active in mind, and your mind – and body – will fail.

Studies show that by the time you are 70 you will have lost about 250 million brain cells. They disappear at the rate of 10,000 a day, and, with age, the parts of the brain that deal with short-term memory (the hippocampi) start to shrink too. But we also know that if you try to improve your memory, there is an increased blood flow to that part of the brain, and US research has found that people who exercise their brains, through playing musical instruments, doing crossroads, reading and playing board games, can reduce their risk of developing dementia. The more challenging the activity, the better. So time to start now, I think. Chess, anyone?

Use mental arithmatic Don't always rely on your calculator or the sales till at the checkout.

Play memory games Time yourself: how fast you can remember the names of 20 flowers, trees, people you know, makes of cars, hits of the 80s and so on?

Log onto the internet for an endless source of puzzles on brain-teasing websites such as www.thinks.com or www.buzancentres.com

Listen to classical music Susan Greenfield, a world expert on the brain, claims it raises your IQ.

Start texting If you're not already into the word-minimizing method on your mobile phone, try it now. Think about different ways to shorten words so your message is quicker to type in. Classic examples include: for=4; to you=2U; before=B4; are you=RU.

Take up bridge A memory for cards is vital.

A great stretch for your spine This yoga position is one of my favourites and very relaxing. Kneel on the floor, sitting on your heels, stretch your arms straight out in front of you and bend forward until your forehead rests on the floor too. Breathe in slowly and out.

Serenity soak Run a deep bath and add three drops each of lavender, frankincense and vetiver essential oil.

Release tension in your neck Sit back comfortably in a chair and lift your shoulders right up to your ears. Hold for a few seconds, and lower again. Repeat three or four times. Then, to help free the neck, rock your head gently from side to side.

Relax Lie on your back, arms by your sides, palms facing upwards. Focus on your breathing, telling yourself you feel warm and peaceful. Be aware of the weight of your body as it grows greater and greater, limb by limb, until you feel unable to move. Concentrate on your breathing for about 5 minutes, and then, when you are ready, wriggle your toes and fingers, open your eyes and get up slowly.

Inhale Add two or three drops of sweetly scented, balancing geranium essential oil to a little warm water in a bowl and leave to diffuse into the air. Or a couple of drops on a tissue to inhale and calm.

Relax your jaw We hold a lot of tension in the jaw without realizing it. Pretend that you're chewing a large toffee very slowly to relieve tension.

f a s t track.

Never a dull moment Stimulate your brain by puzzling out the well-known phrases behind these cryptic clues. For answers, see page 255.

1. Not Guilty Stander
2. gegs
3. m ce m ce m ce
4. O–ER–T–O–
5. tunnelight
6. THOUDEEPGHT
7. ci ii
8. poCARPnd

Laugh Put on a favourite comedy video. Sit back, have hysterics and feel your tension melt away. Laughter also stimulates circulation and helps to boost the immune system by triggering the release of the antibody immunoglobulin A. It supports that most basic theory of wellbeing: if something feels good, it will do you good.

Calm down quickly Breathe in as slowly as you can (aim for a count of 10), and then breathe out equally slowly.

Calm your senses and enliven the mind with a Shiatsu massage technique. Press firmly on the fleshy part of both ears, working from the lower lobe upwards. Repeat once. Then, starting mid-forehead, lightly press your fingertips along your eyebrows, into your temples, behind the ears and down to the nape of your neck.

Energize and relax with a power walk Go on – get out in the fresh air for 20 minutes or longer (see chapter 2).

Hard to sleep? Try this soporific aromatherapy blend. Add two drops of frankincense pure essential oil and one drop each of lavender, marjoram and sandalwood oils to 10ml almond carrier oil. Massage on the neck and chest and breathe in the vapour.

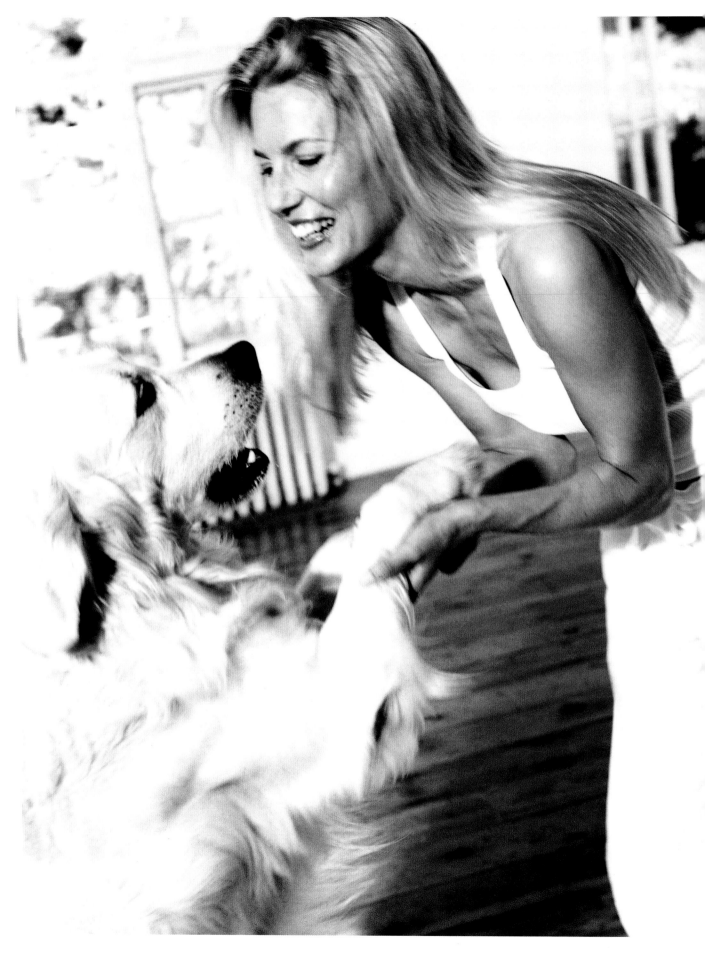

keeping it going

Coping with stress
Which technique will you resort to when a stressful situation arises? If there was one technique you found particularly useful, continue with it. If none, practise them all some more. And use your deep-breathing ritual to help you wind down to sleep after a busy, brain-aching day.

Try to break the mould
You have begun to understand yourself better. Work at recognizing how you deal with situations. If you're an introvert, you tend to get a real sense of self-worth from personal achievement. Extroverts, on the other hand, tend to define themselves in relation to others. Becoming more aware of your responses can help to guide you when making quick judgements and long-term decisions.

Unite mind, body and spirit
● Maintain those breathing rituals and, if you haven't already, try a class in yoga or meditation, pilates or t'ai chi. These deep-breathing mind/body exercises with their energizing effects are mind absorbing, rather than physically exhausting or straining.
● Practise your favourite form of daily massage – for your face, hands, feet, scalp – anything you can easily do for yourself.
● Introduce aromatherapy into every aspect of your life.

Your mind is your sanctuary
Maintain the wind-down moments that work for you. Your mind can become a place of peace and tranquillity when you need it – somewhere to reflect on your emotions and discover a new sense of self.

Seek balance
Keep that new-found calm in every aspect of your life. So remember: organize, prioritize and say no. Make time for your partner – sex is a great stress-buster – and for relaxation.

Choose a better path
● Eat and drink wisely (see chapter 1). Your body needs nutritional reserves to be able to cope with high levels of stress, and any anxiety will be worse if you don't take care of physical health and wellbeing.
● Exercise regularly (see chapter 2). You don't need to do a lot, though it can be habit forming. A daily brisk walk will keep you in good health. But the fitter you are, the better you will feel about yourself.

Hold your head high
Stress affects your posture. Aim to stand, sit and move in a relaxed fashion. Learn the Alexander technique: you immediately become more graceful, elegant and elongated, which must be good for the body. Poor posture says poor self-image so head up, shoulders down, breathe from your abdomen and relax.

Indulge yourself

It treats the soul as well as the body. Whether it's a French manicure, a relaxing facial massage, a deep-conditioning hair treatment or an aromatherapy bath, give yourself a regular pampering session that makes you feel as good as you look. Visit a health spa. Buy flowers for yourself – instead of everyone else. Read that book you've had on your shelves for so long.

Socialize

Join a group, and meet new people who inspire you and make you feel part of something. A loving partner, parents or a circle of close friends are also therapeutic. Positive relationships – hey, even your cat – increase your levels of oxytocin, the anti-stress hormone, so you cope better with testing situations.

Be creative with your time

Time doesn't stand still and neither should you. Expand your mind and your life with new experiences. Take classes in salsa, learn a language or a musical instrument, or start painting.

Spend time just being

Give your mind some time to itself. Find 20–30 minutes for yourself every day. Take a short walk, have a warm bath, a relaxing flower tea, such as camomile, or play some gentle relaxing music.

Seek happiness

Many of us confuse pleasure or contentment with happiness. Pleasure is the next pay cheque, the next holiday, chocolates and wine. You can be a pleasure junkie, always seeking the next fix, but all these experiences are transient. Contentment is long term – being satisfied with your home, your job, your partner. Neither of them is that thing we call happiness or joy.

It is not an emotion: it is a way of being, available to everybody. It is not found in things: it is found in us. Just as the sun is always shining somewhere but we don't see it, so life experiences and our limiting beliefs cloud the happiness that we were born with.

Things that give life meaning increase your chances of finding happiness. They include feeling connected to others and having an active spiritual or religious life. Living in the present, rather than dwelling on past loss or on a real or imagined future, is also a factor. And happiness is far more accessible if you are not constantly seeing yourself in a negative light.

The good news is that, although your happiness quotient is probably influenced by your genes and upbringing, it can be changed for the better. Learn to cope with life events and stress, to feel more in control, and to develop your self-esteem, and you increase your chances of finding happiness.

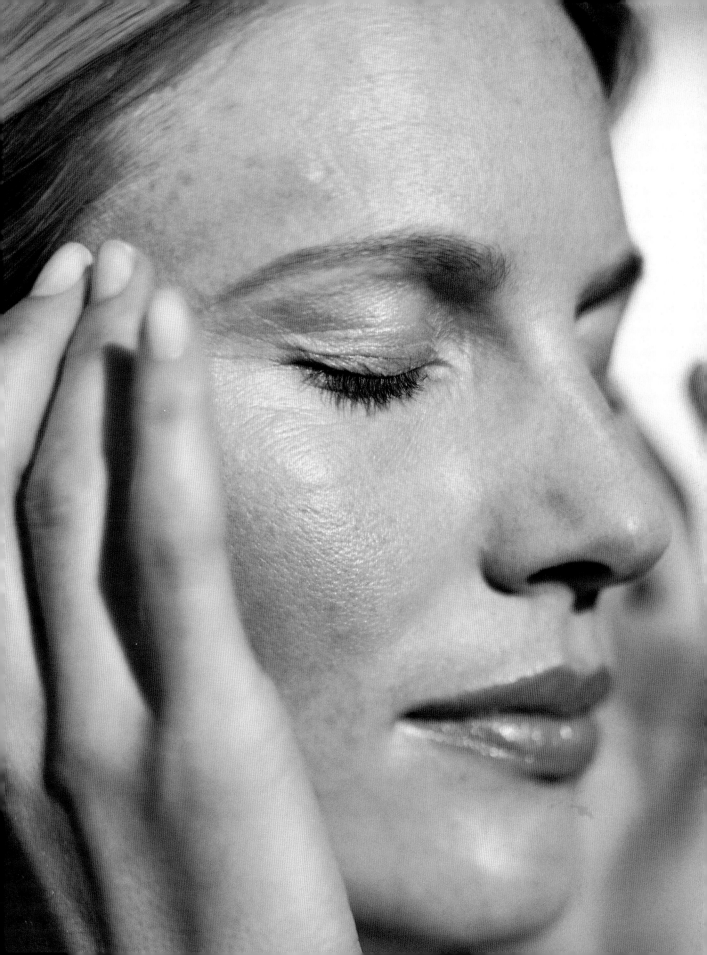

FOCUS
ON THE
NEW YOU

You've achieved – not everything maybe but you've gained more self-knowledge than you know. Value the new you, and you can in time be whatever you want.

reviewing

Great. You've reached day 21. You made a commitment, and you've honoured it. How did you do?

The best way to assess for yourself how much you really gained from the 21-day plan – how much you achieved and how much you need to do it again soon – is to assess your goals. How many can you honestly say you achieved?

If you can tick between 10-15 of the goals listed opposite, you really responded to the whole plan and were totally up for it from the start. You'll benefit hugely from the Top-up Plans on page 238 onwards, and by maintaining elements of the plan into your everyday life.

If you can tick between 5-9 of the goals listed opposite, pat yourself on the back and feel proud of your achievements. It was tough in places, and maybe some aspects of the plan you didn't really enjoy, but you got to grips with it in the end and are beginning to reap the benefits of developing the new you. Try to keep the elements that you enjoyed going to help entice you back in three months' time.

If you can tick between 1-4 of the goals listed opposite, it's time to really treat and pamper yourself. You've done wonderfully well. It wasn't easy, but you've learned so much about yourself – what you want to achieve and where your priorities are in life. View the last 21 days as the start of the new you. Take a break, and then begin the plan again in four to six weeks' time.

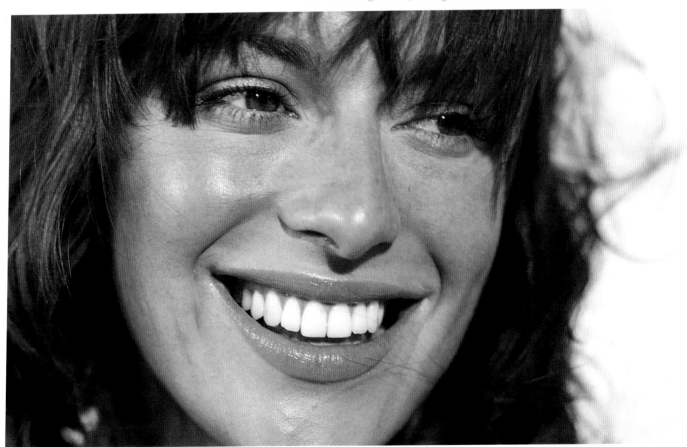

Your nutrition goal

TO TURN AROUND ALL THOSE BAD EATING
HABITS BY IMPROVING YOUR DAILY DIET

Did you..?

☐ Cut out coffee, tea, alcohol and sugary foods?
☐ Bounce out of bed in the morning, feeling energized and looking so much brighter and lighter in yourself?
☐ Change your attitude to food and re-educate your taste buds?

Your fitness goal

TO ESTABLISH AN ACHIEVABLE FITNESS REGIME
THAT REALLY DOES FIT IN WITH YOUR BUSY LIFE

Did you..?

☐ Exercise daily? *Even just for 20 minutes?*
☐ Stretch daily? *Learning your yoga moves well enough not to refer to this book while stretching?*
☐ Look leaner and feel fitter from within?

Your body/skincare goal

TO ILLUMINATE AND SMOOTH YOUR SKIN FROM
WITHIN (FOLLOWING YOUR NUTRITION PLAN
CLOSELY SHOULD HAVE MADE THIS MUCH EASIER)

Did you..?

☐ Get supple, softer skin? Were previous areas of dryness and dehydration made better?
☐ Learn to be more aware of, and love, your body and yourself more?
☐ Take ten years off your looks from top to toe?

Your beauty goal

TO LOOK BETTER GROOMED EACH DAY THROUGH
AN EFFECTIVE HAIR AND MAKE-UP REGIME

Did you..?

☐ Master any new hair styling and make-up techniques?
☐ Update your looks?
☐ Feel more modern and confident in the way you present yourself?

Your low-stress goal

TO FIND MOMENTS TO CONTEMPLATE YOURSELF
AND YOUR LIFE - BOTH GOALS AND PERSONAL
ACHIEVEMENTS - SO ENHANCING EVERY OTHER
ASPECT OF THE PLAN

Did you?

☐ Use the various breathing exercises to help you relax and unwind or focus and recharge?
☐ Learn how to manage your time to suit your life, finding more room for the factors that make you happy, such as family and friendships?
☐ Develop a more positive attitude towards yourself, and others, and life?

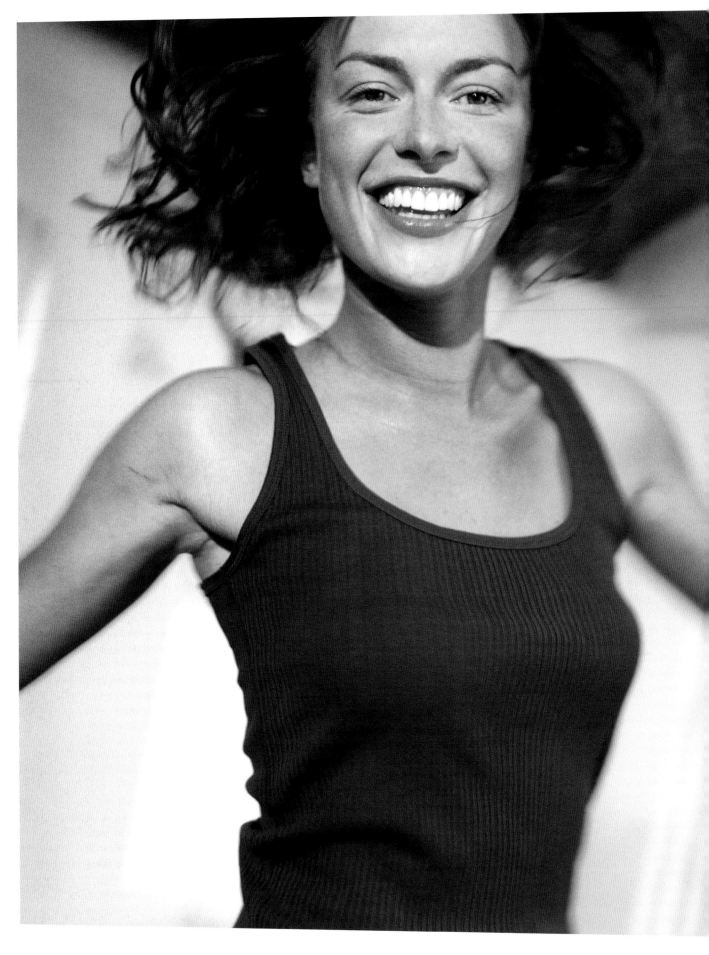

what you have achieved

A shapelier, lighter you	Better grooming
A fitter, healthier body	More time – for you
Better, brighter-looking skin	More control of your life
More energy	A delay to ageing

Now you can see and feel the benefits of healthy eating, regular exercise and a fabulous beauty regime, it's worth noting all the improvements that you've made to spur you on to continue now – or the next time you need a new-you break.

Look back over your notebook if you kept one. Remind yourself how you have changed over the past three weeks – your physique, your attitude and your energy levels. Marvel at the fact that you did it all yourself with just a little will power. You can't give up now. Why would you want to lose that feeling? See this page as an inspiration. Everything here should remind you how far you've come and how much more you can achieve.

A shaplier, lighter you You know now that everything you put in your body reflects on the outside. And you've hopefully experienced the satisfaction of losing your craving for sugary snacks. But it doesn't take much to succumb so always ensure there are plenty of healthy snacks and fresh fruit and vegetables within easy reach.

A fitter, healthier body This is just the start. The fitter you are, the healthier you will be and the better you will feel about yourself. Your daily brisk walk will keep you in good health, but aim to vary with new aerobic exercises or you'll soon tire of it.

Better, brighter looking skin You can now see and feel the difference that comes from thinking about what you put on your skin and into your body. Keep that balance working for you as the ultimate anti-ageing strategy.

More energy You've learned that your body needs nutritional reserves to be able to cope with high levels of stress during a long day – and that stress will only get worse if you don't take care of your physical health and wellbeing. Continue to eat regular meals throughout the day, drink 2 litres (3 ½pt) of water a day and restrict your alcohol intake, limiting yourself to two drinks max in an evening out. Bump up with juices, water and tonic (it looks like a 'drink').

Better grooming You'll find you instinctively know how to make more of your looks/appearance, using hair, make-up, skincare and bodycare tips and advice. Getting ready now seems effortless.

Time for you Creating 'moments' throughout a day just for you is therapy for the mind and soul.

More control of your life The lesson learned is that not everything's perfect – some things take a lot of work from within, discovering how to cope with stress and life events. Happiness is more accessible if you have high self-esteem than if you constantly put yourself down and see yourself in a negative light. .

A delay to ageing Everything you eat and drink, how much sleep you get, how much stress you have in your life, how much exercise you take, together with what you put on your skin, will determine how you age. So use your 21-day plan as a constant support to becoming, and remaining, a new improved you.

maintaining

Learn something new Take up a class in a subject that broadens your mind and your body. Fact is: it doesn't matter what you choose, provided you use this time to explore new interests and focus more on pleasures for you alone.

Pace yourself Remember that we each have an optimum level at which our bodies benefit from exercise. No need to overdo it.

Get yourself a trainer Even if you opt for just a course of six sessions, the intense experience of a personal trainer will give you a new outlook on your Fitness regime – and introduce more variety to ensure that you don't lose interest. Remember that motivation is the key to keeping fit.

See a colour consultant A professional consultant can help you determine which colours suit you best, and thereby slim down your wardrobe into styles and colours that flatter the way you look now. Don't be a slave to this regime. Simply be inspired by what works for you.

Arrange a pampering treat once a month Whether it's reflexology, aromatherapy massage, reiki, pedicure or a facial, show your body how much you care by nurturing it with love and attention from all sources. And keep it up at home. Set yourself an hour every three days to devote to a mask, pedicure or manicure...whatever makes you feel good.

Focus on your goals Choose one and concentrate purely on that for a month. Then add another the next month and so on. Having a personal goal – whether it's for nutrition, fitness or beauty – will boost your motivation and can make you feel more confident and self-assured.

Relax regardless You can resolve so many problems and anxieties with a calmer approach to life. Practise deep breathing, meditation and visualization until they become second nature. Seek out classes if you find it hard to manage on your own. Relaxation techniques are the best way to get control of your life, and the means are totally within your power.

Live a little Accept setbacks to your new regime, such as dining out, major celebrations, illness and so on. Being fit and healthy is a 'life style' – a style for life. Setbacks are normal so accept that it's OK to stray every now and then, provided you come back with even more enthusiasm.

Reminders

KEEP THIS LIST WITH YOU WHEREVER YOU GO – IN THE CAR, IN YOUR HANDBAG, BY THE FRIDGE, AS A BOOKMARK. CHECK IT CONSTANTLY – TO HELP REINFORCE THE PLAN TODAY AND BEYOND.

● I am drinking 2 litres of water a day – herbal teas and fruit juices count to a point.

● I have a healthy relationship with food. I eat to fuel my body with energy.

● Food sustains me and makes me feel happier about myself. Sugar brings me down. I eat regularly, three times a day, to keep my blood-sugar levels stable and reduce my cravings.

● I don't need stimulants. Cigarettes, coffee, tea or alcohol are occasional treats in my life – I do not need them on a regular basis.

● Exercise makes me feel happier in myself. I need to exercise 20 minutes every day.

● When I close my eyes and hear nothing, I can think about nothing that bothers me – only happiness and peace.

● I am content. My life isn't perfect – but that would be dull. I don't seek perfection, only contentment.

● I am proud of who I am and what I am. I love myself. I love and am loved.

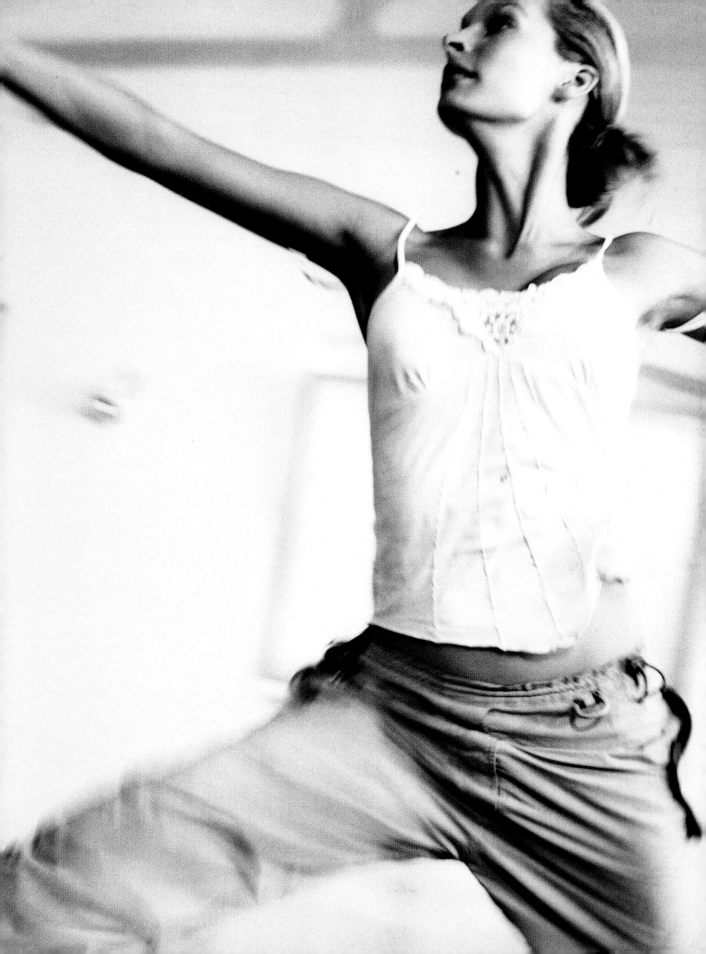

YOUR
THREE
TOP-UP
PLANS

Use these short programmes to boost all the work you've done whenever you get the chance. Once you get the hang of things, you can devise your own...

weekend spa programme

Got a whole precious weekend to yourself? Take time to focus on many of the mind/body pampering treatments and rituals from the 21-day plan. Come Monday morning you'll feel so good, you'll be inclined to start the 21 days again...

OK, so the most important aspect of this weekend spa programme is that you devote the whole time to you and you alone. No partners, girlfriends or children are allowed. This is your time. Each day is organized so you glide from one session to another. And for those moments when there's free time with nothing particularly planned, choose relaxing, de-stressful things to do. There's no TV, newspapers or radio. But there is that fabulous novel you've been meaning to finish, mind puzzles and games such as word searches or crosswords, learning how to play chess with the computer, power naps and, of course, relaxing feel-good music (but preferably nothing too staccato!).

Your spa programme needs

Make your spa weekend go as smoothly and unstressfully as possible by planning ahead. Have everything you need to hand, and stock up the day before you begin on fresh foods.

A light menu Choose your menus from days 3–7 of the Nutrition programme: these are the lightest, most cleansing part of the regime. Get plenty of fresh fruit, 'coloured' vegetables, salad stuff, nuts, rice cakes, live yoghurt, fruit smoothies, lemons (for hot-water drinks) and herbal teas to drink through the day.

Mud & marine ingredients Do you have everything you need? You are going to focus on home treatments that help to boost the detoxing effect of your eating programme: the detoxifying mud wrap, deep-sea soak and deep-cleansing face mask. Coupled with hot water and lemon drinks and plenty of fresh mineral water, you'll feel cleansed inside and out.

Body pleasures Check those manicure and pedicure bits, the aromatherapy oils (to wake-up and relax you in the bath and in the air), the luscious oil & salt scrub, fake tan and your body brush. Over these two days you can dramatically boost the colour and condition of the skin on your body.

Facial wonders Treats in store include a face scrub, choice of face mask, everything for the basic skincare regime, facial massage oil or serum, and a facial steam. If you've been under a great deal of stress, it is especially important to focus on facial regimes that boost and revitalize your skin.

Heavenly hair You must have everything you need for the basic shampoo & conditioning regime, but what about a conditioning hair mask? No hairdryer required – you're in for a weekend of pampering, so give 'pandering to perfection' a miss.

For fitness Get out that loose/stretchy clothing, your trainers and a mat. Short, 20-minute bursts of exercise followed by body revitalizing treatments only benefit your spa programme further.

Don't miss Water. Hopefully I've said it for the last time, but you can hardly have too much of it this weekend. It's nature's natural tranquillizer, a must for the complete mind, body and soul.

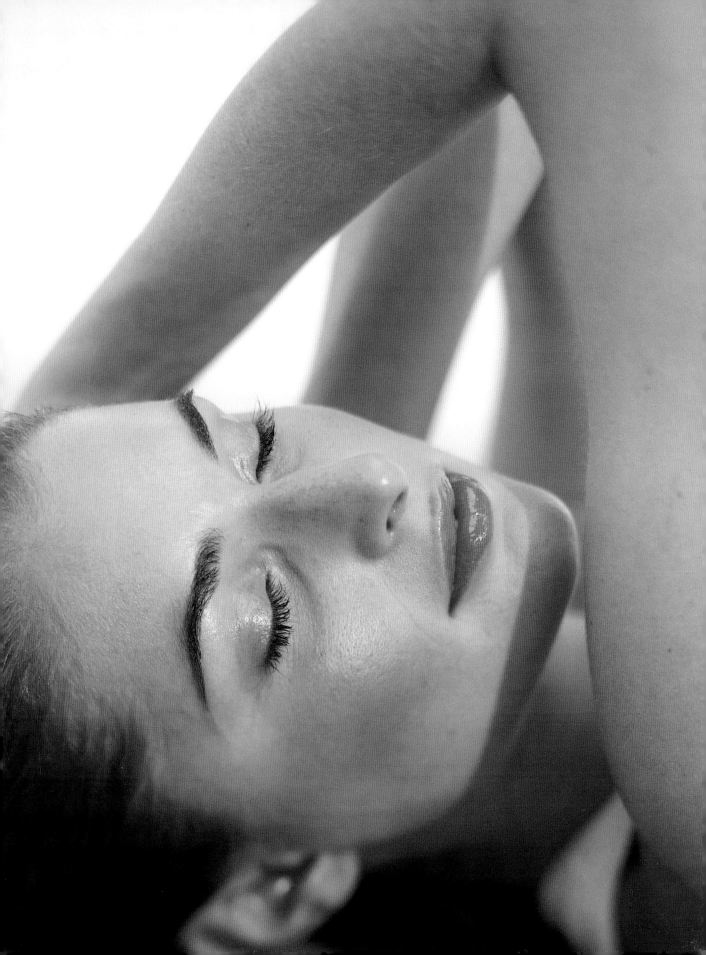

Your weekend spa planner

Friday

6.30pm	Herbal tea
7.00pm	Supper (see day 3–7 menus)
8.00pm	Pamper pedicure ☆
8.20pm	Affirmations
8.30pm	Facial scrub ♡
8.45pm	Cleansing facial mask ♡
8.50pm	Skincare (pm) regime
9.00pm	with anti-ageing facial massage ☆
9.30pm	Aromatherapy (relaxing bath) ☆
10.00pm	Wind-down moments
	with breathing ritual ☆

Saturday

	Hot water & lemon
6.30am	Wake-up moment (aromatherapy)
6.50am	Early-morning stretch
7.00am	Oil & salt scrub ♡
7.10am	Body (am) regime
7.20am	Skin (am) regime
7.30am	Breakfast (see day 3–7 menus)
9.00am	Scalp massage ♡
9.30am	Conditioning hair mask ♡
11.00am	Body fake tan ☆
11.30am	Energy smoothie while tan develops
12.00am	Midday moments
12.30pm	Lunch
1.00pm	Midday aerobics (walk)
2.00pm	Power nap
3.00pm	Deep-sea soak ♡
4.00pm	Rest & relax (restorative moment)
4.30pm	Mind power (visualization) ☆
5.00pm	Energy smoothie
6.30pm	Evening tone-up
7.00pm	Supper
8.00pm	Quick body-smoothing wrap ♡
8.30pm	Body (pm) regime
9.00pm	Skin (pm) regime
9.30pm	Breathing ritual ☆
10.00pm	Wind-down moments

Sunday

	Hot water & lemon
6.30am	Wake-up moment (aromatherapy)
6.50am	Early-morning stretch
7.00am	Body (am) regime
7.10am	Face-mapping session ☆
7.20am	Facial steam ♡
7.30am	Deep-cleansing facial mask ♡
9.00am	Skin (am) regime
9.30am	Breakfast (see day 3–7 menus)
10.00am	Hair regime
11.00am	Blow-dry ♡
11.30am	Energy smoothie
12.30pm	Lunch
1.00pm	Midday aerobics (walk)
2.00pm	Power nap
3.00pm	Detoxifying mud wrap ♡
4.00pm	Mind power (meditation) ☆
4.30pm	Energy smoothie
5.00pm	Manicure ☆
6.30pm	Rest & relax (as polish dries)
7.00pm	Supper
8.30pm	Foot massage ☆
9.00pm	Body (pm) regime
9.30pm	Skin (pm) regime
10.00pm	Wind-down moments

I've shown times in script because they are your choice. ♡ represents a beautifier and ☆ a booster.

The times are approximate –
it's your weekend after all – but they are a good guide. Adapt the planner however you wish, and feel free to repeat or replace favourite treatments or sessions. Just enjoy...

Don't skimp
The number one tip for gorgeous body skin is to moisturize. Massage in plenty of body cream or body oil after every bathing treatment to avoid dehydration and to keep your skin gleaming. Spend 10–15 minutes, massaging your body with upward strokes from the feet to the thighs, from the hands to the shoulders, as you do in body brushing.

Your goal is to recharge yourself in little more than 48 hours. So take the phone off the hook and don't answer the door. You'll find this weekend has the same benefit as a week's holiday.

Your aim is to energize, calm, brighten, treat and cleanse inside and out.

Perfect for times when you've been overdoing things – work, food, alcohol – or have really slipped from the routine established during the 21-day plan. Frequent breaks from your everyday lifestyle will help to remind you about the principles of the complete programme.

Focus on ways to rewind and recharge body and soul. Treat this time as if you really were spending a weekend in a spa. Make the most of all the bodycare rituals in particular – the deep-sea soak, the blissful bathing ritual, the detoxifying mud wrap, and so on. Rest at intervals during the day, especially after a treatment. This can be extremely invigorating but it also feels wonderfully indulgent. And that's what you need to get from this spa weekend, the feeling that you've devoted real quality time to yourself.

What you'll achieve

● *Self-worth* Setting aside time for yourself in this way, on a regular basis, will enhance both physical and psychological wellbeing, equally vital if you are to maintain a more positive attitude to yourself. It's not enough to squeeze your pampering into tiny occasional time slots. You MUST make time – a set amount of time – even if it's only one day instead of two. And don't feel guilty about it. You matter.
● *Body confidence* It's one of the most attractive assets you can possess. When you feel good about yourself, everyone else feels it too. Your positive nature illuminates your inner life, and others thrive on your company. And that feels good.

Rest and relaxation

● Choose 10 minutes here and 10 minutes there for quiet, peaceful moments to light a few candles and meditate, to snuggle up under a duvet and read, or to listen to music – all to recreate that 'spa lounge' feel.

● Make the most of your solitude with the relaxation technique you used first in the blissful bath ritual. Remember you need something to rest your head on as you lie back, close your eyes, and breathe slowly and evenly in and out to a count of 4. Concentrate on releasing the tensions in your body as you work from your head down to your feet. Then let your head fill with the white light that represents everything warm, good and positive in your life. Wrap it around any negative thoughts that come into your mind until there's only a sense of peace left behind.

Aromatherapy energizer

Mix two drops each of grapefruit, lemon and rosemary essential oils together. Either add to the bath water, step in and immerse yourself in the fragrant warm water for 20 minutes or add to a vaporizer (or bowl of hot water) and inhale instead.

hot date programme

When you've a couple of hours to get ready for a great night out with a new love, old flame, loving partner or just good friends, a set of fabulous, instant beautifiers and boosters will make you feel so much more confident. And knowing what you have time for alleviates the stress of getting ready too.

Your golden rule for getting your look right and being on time is simply that old maxim 'less is more'. Perhaps you're going out soon after work? Loading on the foundation, colourful blusher and bold lipstick in the belief that it's going to make you look less tired or younger, just doesn't work. Treat this time as if you're at a salon getting ready for a big night out. Make the most of all the beauty rituals – the evening make-up regime, manicure, pedicure – all the things that make you feel good from the outside in. Since you've already completed the 21-day plan, you should feel more confident about applying make-up and the way it can make you look.

Your hot-date programme needs

Check you have everything you need to hand before the evening so you can be ready and gorgeous with the minimum of stress.

Flawless skin things It's the basic skin (am) regime, and then prep with a special under make-up skin-smoothing beauty essence or radiance cream. These light, textured gels contain silicone polymers that create a smoother surface for make-up and blur expression lines so wrinkles appear less pronounced.

A youthful make-up kit The essentials are: foundation or concealer, applied only where you need it; a shimmery pale eyeshadow that acts as an all-over shadow to banish redness or darkness on the eyes, takes seconds to apply and requires little expertise; every girl's eyeliner – liquid, cake, powder or pencil – to enhance the shape of your eyes (see page 158 to remind yourself how); totally essential mascara; a pinky beige lip-toned liner, softened with a sheer or berry-toned lipgloss to lightly define; and warm blusher to add a flattering blush to the cheeks.

A smooth shimmery body Check out ingredients for the oil & salt scrub that will leave your skin so delicious. You'll follow up with a shower rather than a soak and you can swap your usual moisturizer for a golden body glow – glistening lotion or oil with shimmery particles, perfect for making skin look sexy.

Manicure & pedicure bits This has to be the quickest way to add glamour: condition, moisturize and polish to perfection.

A chic hair-do So it's your basic shampoo and conditioner – plus a conditioning hair mask if your hair is long – and time to blow-dry smooth if you can. Smoother hair is shinier and looks more groomed. Style it up or leave it down, whichever you prefer.

Easy-wear wardrobe Choose something simple in a style you feel comfortable in. Beware of exposing the midriff if yours is less than toned. Choose a skirt length that flatters your height and shape, and heel heights you can cope with.

Don't miss There are things you don't ever do before a hot date: never try out a new face mask, facial steam or anything that your skin's not used to. You may get a reaction.

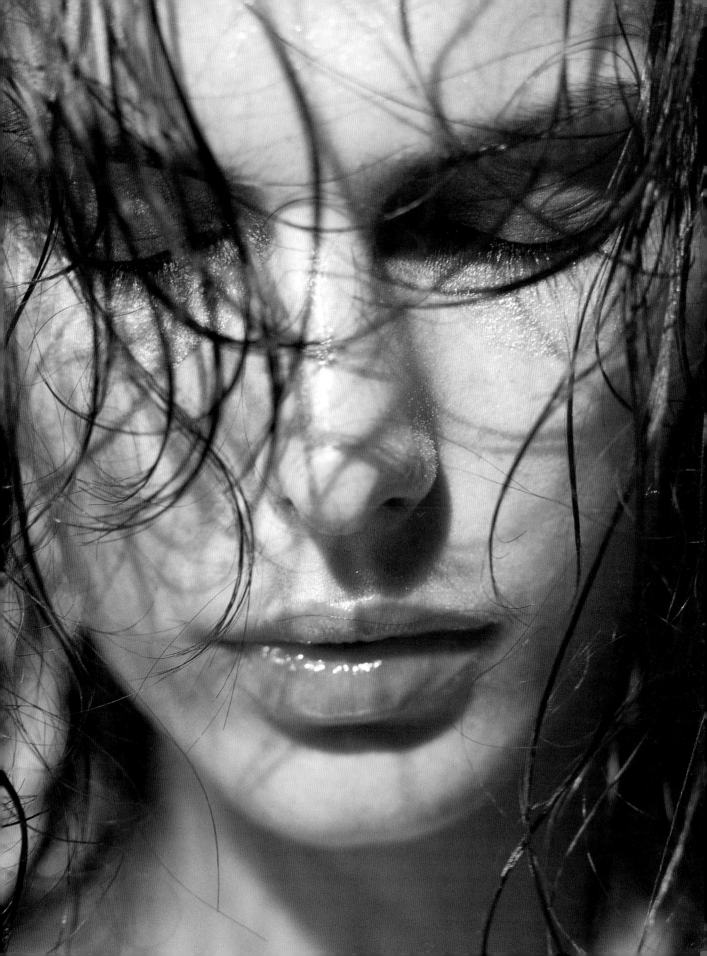

Your hot date planner

Time	Routine
6.00pm	Repeat the morning shower from the Body (am) regime, replacing the dry body brushing with a oil & salt scrub
6.15pm	Your body won't need moisturizer now so apply a golden, skin-glistening lotion instead if you have one to hand
6.25pm	Shampoo and condition your hair Use an intensive conditioning treatment if it's medium to long
6.35pm	Blow-dry with volume
7.00pm	Breathing ritual: to recharge
7.10pm	Repeat the Skincare (am) regime if there's time; otherwise spritz your skin with a facial spray or toner, pat dry and apply a radiance cream
7.20pm	Dress. Go for simple – it's more stunning (Get your keys out of your bag and ready by the door)
7.25pm	Pedicure & manicure: use a speed-dry top coat, and drink your smoothie while the polish dries
7.45pm	Make-up for night, emphasizing your eyes or your lips (Take care not to smudge your nails as you go)
8.00pm	Get into cab

I've shown times in script because they are your choice.

Aromatherapy energiser

Make sure you add an essential oil to your shower, diluted in 50ml water. Choose stimulating pure rosemary or citrus oils, such as grapefruit, tangerine or lemon. Maintain the therapy by sprinkling two drops of a favourite oil onto a tissue and inhaling as you get ready, or vaporize around your home.

Refresh and energize

● Use your breathing ritual to clear your mind and help focus on what you want to achieve in these two hours (see page 214).

●Make yourself an energy treat. A fresh fruit smoothie packed full of goodness and energy will pick you up when you need to keep going. Don't turn to alcohol to put you in the party mood – it's a depressant.

Your goal is to look just incredible without keeping anyone waiting.

Your aim is to use every invitation as an opportunity to practise those newly acquired beauty skills until they take no time at all.

Perfect for times when you're due to go out, but don't really feel 'in the mood'. This mini regime will refresh you so you're ready to party.

Focus on ways to refresh and re-energize yourself from top to toe after a long day. Spritz your favourite perfume, smooth on an aromatic, invigorating body cream, massage your toes, refresh your hair (see page 197). And practise make-up techniques that will enhance your features. The most dramatic evening make-up is one that gives your face a single focal point – emphasizing either your eyes or your lips (see pages 158 and 160 for tips). Keep make-up light. You add ten years if you make it heavy; you take ten years off if you aim for sheer and lightweight.

What you'll achieve

● *Casual elegance* Having everything you need to hand will help to ensure that you stick to a regime that works for you. The end result is make-up that takes less time to apply and creates natural good looks with ease.

● *Renewed confidence* Looking good will boost your self-esteem. But it works both ways: you need to feel good to look good too. Practising beauty regimes that enhance your looks can only have a positive effect on the way you think and feel about yourself and your body.

Don't skimp Give yourself time. Be prepared for last-minute chaos, from that broken fingernail, end-of-day exhaustion and bad-hair moment to smudged make-up. The earlier you start, the more relaxed and pampered you'll feel.

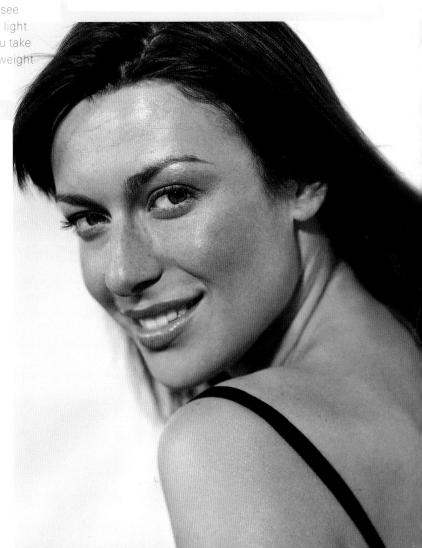

special occasion programme

For those times when a camera points in your direction, for a wedding, christening, celebratory birthday or party, or simply a last-minute holiday abroad, this 5-day special programme will shape your silhouette enough for you to start feeling lighter and lovelier.

You want to slink into something prettier than usual – to dress yourself up and look your best. Well, it helps if you focus on the inside too. In effect, you'll be cramming the whole of the first week of the 21-day plan into just five days. It's going to be busy, but try to fit in as many of the treatments as possible. The more you do, the more likely you are to achieve your goal by day 5. However, if it's a really special occasion – if you're a bridesmaid (after all the bride always looks her best), mother of the bride, going on a romantic weekend or on a beach holiday), I'd be inclined to do the whole 21 days again if you have the time, or at least days 10–14 as well, by which time you will really feel lighter and brighter in every way.

Your programme needs

On the run up to any special occasion you have to plan ahead. Make sure you have everything you need in advance to make these five days easier.

A lighter menu The meals on days 3 to 7 are the lightest, and the hardest, days in the original Nutrition programme. It's detox time so you know the drill. You need to stock up on fresh fruit, 'coloured' vegetables, salad stuff, nuts, rice cakes, lemons, mineral water and those herbal teas.

Body treats From massage to scrubs, soaks to wraps, pedicure to manicure, lemon oil to lemon water, make sure you're well prepared. Your body will love the attention and you are going to love the effect.

Fitness Get out the loose/stretchy clothing (for running and stretching), your trainers and a mat. You've experienced how just 20 minutes of daily exercise combined with body revitalizing treatments can boost the feel-good/look-good factor.

Fabulous facials You'll be treating your skin to plenty of pampering scrubs and masks, as well as a complete home facial and a massage, so make a detailed checklist. My hope is that you'll be able to fit everything into your busy week, while feeling that you've really treated yourself.

Better grooming It's the hair and make-up must-haves again. But use this time to experiment too – styling both your hair and your make-up for the big occasion. Turn to chapters 5 and 6 for tips and advice.

Don't miss Try to take time off if you can. The more positive vibes you can get from the various therapies and mind-power techniques, the better.

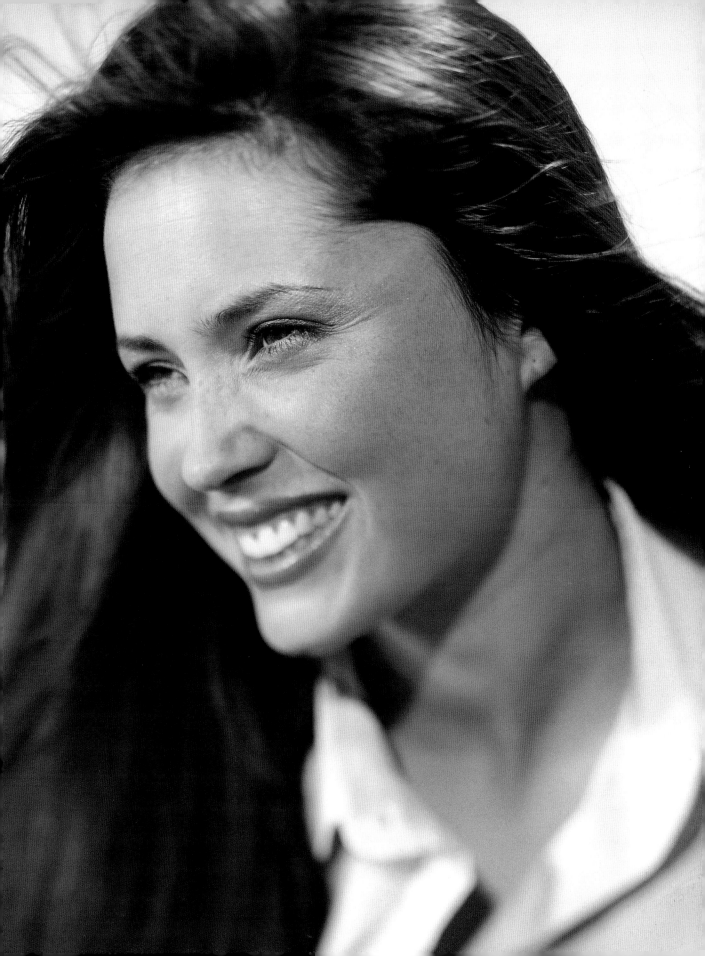

Your special occasion planner

Day 1

6.20am	Wake-up moments
6.40am	Hot water & lemon
6.50am	Morning feel-good stretch ☆
7.00am	Oil & salt scrub ♡
7.10am	Facial scrub ♡
7.20am	Skin (am) regime
7.30am	Breakfast (see day 3 menu)
7.45am	Hair regime
8.00am	Conditioning hair mask ♡
8.15am	Blow-dry ♡
11.00am	Energy smoothie
12.00am	Midday moments
12.30am	Midday aerobics
1.00pm	Lunch
	Mind power (games) ☆
6.30pm	Evening tone-up
7.00pm	Supper
8.30pm	Deep-sea soak ♡
9.00pm	Body (pm) regime
9.45pm	Skin (pm) regime
	with anti-ageing facial massage ☆
10.15pm	Wind-down moments
	with breathing ritual ☆

Day 2

6.20am	Wake-up moments
6.40am	Hot water & lemon
6.50am	Morning feel-good stretch ☆
7.00am	Body (am) regime
7.10am	Facial mask ♡
7.20am	Skin (am) regime
7.30am	Breakfast (see day 4 menu)
7.45am	Brow shaping ☆
11.00am	Energy smoothie
12.00am	Midday moments
12.30am	Midday aerobics (walk)
1.00pm	Lunch
	Mind power (meditation) ☆
7.00pm	Supper
8.30pm	Body-smoothing wrap ♡
9.00pm	Aromatherapy (relaxing bath) ☆
9.45pm	Skin (pm) regime
10.00pm	Relaxing foot massage ☆
10.15pm	Wind-down moments
	with breathing ritual ☆

Day 3

6.30am	Hot water & lemon
6.40am	Early-morning stretch
7.00am	Body (am) regime
7.10am	Skin (am) regime
7.20am	Breakfast (see day 5 menu)
7.30am	Hair regime
7.45am	Blow-dry ♡
8.15am	Face fake tan ☆
11.00am	Energy smoothie
11.30am	Time management ☆
12.30am	Midday aerobics
1.00pm	Lunch
2.00pm	Affirmations
6.30pm	Evening tone-up
7.00pm	Supper
8.30pm	Body (pm) regime
9.00pm	Manicure ☆
9.45pm	Skin (pm) regime
	with anti-ageing facial massage ☆
10.30pm	Wind-down moments
	with breathing ritual ☆

I've shown times in script because they are your choice. ♡ represents a beautifier and ☆ a booster.

Your goal is to smooth and shape your body in preparation for a special occasion.

Your aim is a great improvement in the way you look and feel, inside and out, in under a week.

Perfect for times when you've got an incentive. Motivation is the key so use the occasion as a way of keeping yourself on track. I'd also recommend doing this mini 5-day programme every two to three months after finishing the 21-day plan. Indeed, if you can plot a few special occasion programmes through your year, you can be sure you will really start to see the long-term benefits of your original 21-day plan – and feel more confident and self-assured about the way you look and feel should such occasions arise.

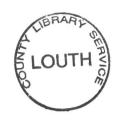

COUNTY LIBRARY SERVICE

LOUTH

Day 4

6.30am	Hot water & lemon
6.40am	Early-morning stretch
7.00am	Oil & salt scrub ♡
7.10am	Skin (am) regime
7.30am	Breakfast (see day 6 menu)
7.45am	Hair regime
11.00am	Energy smoothie
11.30am	Create order ☆
12.30am	Midday aerobics
1.00pm	Lunch
2.00pm	Affirmations
7.00pm	Supper
8.30pm	Detoxifying mud wrap ♡
9.00pm	Aromatherapy (relaxing bath) ☆
9.45pm	Skin (pm) regime
10.00pm	Relaxing facial ☆
10.30pm	Wind-down moments
	with breathing ritual ☆

Day 5

6.20am	Wake-up moments
6.30am	Hot water & lemon
6.40am	Early-morning stretch
7.00am	Body (am) regime
7.20am	Skin (am) regime
7.45am	Breakfast (see day 7 menu)
8.00am	Hair regime
8.15am	Blow-dry ♡
8.25am	Lash curling ☆
11.00am	Energy smoothie
11.30am	Mind power (visualization) ☆
12.00am	Midday moments
1.00pm	Lunch
2.00pm	Midday aerobics
6.30pm	Evening tone-up
7.00pm	Supper
	Deep-sea soak ♡
8.30pm	Body (pm) regime
9.00pm	Pedicure ☆
9.30pm	Skin (pm) regime
	with revitalizing facial mask ♡
10.00pm	Wind-down moments
	with breathing ritual ☆

What you'll achieve

● *Feel-good factor* Check page 28 (end of week one in the Nutrition programme) for a reminder right now. Because you've already done the 21-day programme everything will feel quite familiar and should take far less effort than it did the first time around.

● *A better body* From the inside out and the outside in, you cosset every bit of skin from top to toe, and it shows. You will glow with renewed health and vitality.

● *A positive reminder* A shorter version of the whole 21-day plan will give your mind and body a healthy reminder, and put you back on a better path, hopefully now for life.

Focus on ways to better your body and mind from top to toe. Each day in the programme has a different focus, from relaxing to enhancing, as you build to the final day when you re-emerge feeling refreshed and rejuvenated from a period of healthy eating, body cosseting and no stimulants.

● *Smooth & soften on Day 1.* From your hair (conditioning mask) to your body (oil & salt scrub), you're lavishing oils and creams on your body to improve its condition.

● *Relax and soothe on Day 2.* You're cleansing from within and flexing that body, but a mask and relaxing aromatherapy help you take it easy while the toxins are being eliminated. (Try to have this day off if you can.)

● *Enhance on Day 3.* Manicure, facial fake tan and face massage boost your outer confidence.

● *Refocus on Day 4.* Positive affirmations and mind-power techniques are essential on the fourth day, as they encourage you to make time for your mind as well as your body.

● *Emerge on Day 5.* Preened, bright eyed, clearer of mind, you are far more at one with yourself than you were five days ago.

Index

Answers to the brain-teasing puzzles on page 225

1. Innocent bystander **2**. Scrambled eggs **3**. Three blind mice (no 'i's) **4**. Painless operation **5**. Light at the end of the tunnel
6. Deep in thought **7**. See eye to eye **8**. Big fish in a little pond

Author's acknowledgements

I would especially like to thank my wonderful agent, Fiona Lindsay of Limelight Management, for her endless support and encouragement, and Jane O'Shea at Quadrille Publishing for allowing me write this book in the first place. I would also like to send my love and thanks to Iain Philpott, whose beautiful photography has helped to make this health and beauty programme all the more appealing, and to Richard Sinclair at The Warehouse Studio, SW18, for the location and the loan of Archie, his golden retriever. Thank you, too, to my dear friends Sheena Miller, Catherine Everest, Carolyn Bailey, Nancy Brady, Suzanne Wilson and Kate Harris, who have kept me going throughout. And, of course, my husband, Jim Stanton, and my dear children, Olivia, William and little Phoebe.

Special thanks go to experts: Lee Bradley, Frances and Michael Van Clarke, Mathew Alexander, Beverly Cobella and Denise McAdam for hair, Amanda Birch at Michaeljohn for skin, aromatherapist Glenda Taylor, and Ann Louise Gittleman for her advice on nutrition. And to the wonderful make-up artists on this book: Jenny Dodson and Aimee Adams.

Publisher's acknowledgements

The publisher wishes to thank Margaret Howell for the beautiful clothes, Jo and Nina at Wink Management for their wonderful organization, Finders International for the body mud; Origins for the body scrub; Hildon for their refreshing water, and The White Company.

Picture acknowledgements
The publisher wishes to thank the following organizations for their kind permission to reproduce the following photographs: 24-7, 30–3, 36–9 and 151 right Digital Vision, 151 centre Photodisc/Getty.
All the special photography was by Iain Philpott.